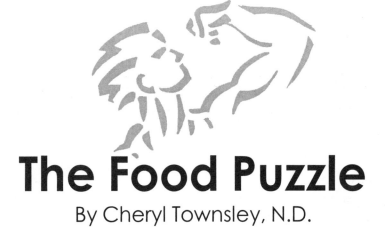

The Food Puzzle

By Cheryl Townsley, N.D.

A LFH Publication • Littleton, Colorado

ISBN 0-9644566-3-X

Graphics: Nick Zellinger
Text Design: Theresa Frank

This publication is designed to provide accurate and authoritative information in regard to the subject matter covered. It is sold with the understanding that the author and the publisher are not engaged in rendering legal, medical or other professional service. If medical services or other expert consultation is required, the services of a competent professional should be sought.

Townsley, Cheryl
  The Food Puzzle™ /
  Cheryl Townsley, N.D.
  1. Nutrition. 2. Health. I. Title.

For information contact:

LFH Publishing
6520 S Broadway
Littleton, CO 80121
303-794-4477
www.lifestyleforhealth.com
email: forest@lifestyleforhealth.com
For ordering information, refer to the last page.

Printed in the United States of America

CONTENTS

ACKNOWLEDGEMENTS

Many people have provided expertise to help me in my research and development of the *Food Puzzle*™. No practitioner can ever develop something that has not been based on the work of others. The following list is only a partial list, as there are many people that I might be unaware of their work in the health field. To those I have overlooked, please accept my appreciation for your efforts.

I appreciate James Balch M.D., Dave Frahm, Bruce Fife N.D., Ray Gebauer, Gordon Tessler PhD., Norman Walker and Bernard Jensen for their extensive work in the basics of nutritional health.

I appreciate the work of Mannatech and Ann Louise Gittleman in their work on metabolic profiling. Anne Louise Gittleman's work has been helpful in many ways, including her understanding of parasites, cleansing and the need for good fats.

I appreciate the work on the glycemic index that was done by the Glycemic Research Institute, Steve Nuggent N.M.D., H. Leighton Steward, Morrison C. Bethea M.D., Sam S. Andrews M.D. and Luis A. Balart M.D. Their work on the impact of high glycemic foods and refined sugar has been outstanding.

I appreciate the work of Brenda Watson C.T., William Crook M.D. and Gail Burton for their extensive work in the area of Candida and Candida cleanses. Brenda Watson has developed excellent products to use for Candida as well as other cleansing protocols.

I appreciate the work of Dr. Peter J. D'Adamo and his ground-breaking studies on the blood type diet. He and his father have extensively studied this topic and brought great insight to the health field on the role of blood type on diet.

Each of these men and women has greatly helped me improve my health and the health of thousands of others. We recognize, acknowledge and express our appreciation for their diligence and commitment to the quest of optimal health.

I appreciate the work and expertise of Howard Loomis, D.C., Dennis Frerking, D.C. and the work of 21st Century in the field of enzyme therapy. The Enzyme Solution product line has greatly benefited clients. Thank you also to Dr. Sandra Fico and her work with Neurosomatic Programming (NSP) which has further supported our work with digestion and reconnecting the brain and various body functions.

I appreciate the Barlean's team (Bruce Barlean, Jade Beutler and Ray Palys) for providing a superior flax product. Forest and I also appreciate their support and expertise in the vision of *Body by Design* as a product and Lifestyle as a business.

Thank you also to my loyal LFH publishing team without which I could never get a book to print. From design, to editing, to marketing, this team is great and I appreciate each of you.

To our LFH Coaches and the new ones to come, I say thank you for carrying the message of wholeness to a nation that faces unparalleled health concerns. Only a team can carry a message to the masses. I appreciate each one of you taking this message to your sphere of influence.

To Forest and Anna I say thank you for being the most special people in my life. I love you and appreciate your support of my destiny and purpose. To my Lord, I say thank you for giving me a destiny and purpose that burns passionately in my heart – *to see people whole to live out their God-given potential.*

INTRODUCTION

Food ... simple yet oh so complex! How can such a simple four-letter word cause such confusion in the United States? Bookstores have entire aisles dedicated to the "right" eating plan. Doctors and health care practitioners promise quick results on the "right" eating plan.

The highly recommended ingredients of one "right" plan are often the "avoid" ingredients of another "right" plan. For example, some experts expound on high protein and low carbohydrates as the only way to effectively lose weight. Others insist that vegetarian and high carbohydrates diets are the only way to build health. Then others simply require eating low-sugar foods. What is the "right" approach to the best foods?

What Makes the Food Puzzle Different?

Customization Based on Wisdom

Over the years one of my favorite words has become *wisdom*. As a child I defined *wisdom* as simply knowing a lot – being smart. As I got a little older I defined *wisdom* as the accumulation of knowledge. Today, after years of working on my own health and the health of thousands of clients, I find those definitions to be accurate, yet incomplete.

I have worked with many clients where the rule for a health situation did not work for them. They were unique and needed a customized solution to fit their specific needs. As a result, I now define *wisdom* as:

"Knowing what question to ask, and of whom, or where to ask that question."

This is a key definition not only for teachers, but also for health care providers. Once a key question is asked of the right source, answers become apparent. Nowhere is this more true than in the area of food. The above question, *"What is the 'right' approach to the best foods?"* is not the question I have learned to ask.

I now ask the question *"What is the best food for this individual to have optimal health and maximum energy?"* That question naturally leads to other questions, including: "What foods compromise health and diminish energy in the individual?" Most experts agree on the basics of the "no-no" foods.

Foods that have no health benefit that need to be eliminated by everybody are:
- white flour and white flour-based products
- white sugar and products that contain white sugar
- white rice
- hydrogenated fats (shortening, vegetable oils, etc.)
- food dyes and preservatives
- ingredient names on labels that you can't pronounce

The removal of these foods is the first place to start in building your customized *Food Puzzle*. If you are currently consuming these foods, you may need to take time to learn how to eliminate them from your diet. Many excellent books are available to help you. I have authored two books, *Food Smart!*

which helps you make the changes on a budget and *Lifestyle for Health Cookbook* which provides over 400 recipes and key strategies to help you implement the plan in the kitchen. Both books are available from Lifestyle for Health or your local health food store. Simply removing the "no-no" foods can cause a significant increase in your energy and health.

Start with the basics that can help anyone. That is the foundation from which we all agree. From that foundation, the *Food Puzzle* will provide you with many ways to customize your plan and truly make it *your plan!*

Customization Based on Research & Common Sense

The *Food Puzzle* has four basic customizing factors to help you customize a plan that works for you instead of trying to make a general plan fit you. Each of these factors has been extensively researched and is highly credited in the health industry.

Those factors include:
1. Metabolic Profiling (the best *ratio* of proteins, fats and carbohydrates for maximum energy)
2. Glycemic Index (blood sugar balancing for balanced hormones and fat burning)
3. Candida (identification of the presence of fungus that can hinder weight loss and create other health issues)
4. Blood Type (the best *source* of proteins, fats and carbohydrates to eat and to avoid, along with unique considerations for exercise and supplementation)

As excellent as the research is for each of these factors, I have found that any of these factors can be used to support unhealthy choices. Let's take a look at how each of these could be used to create an unhealthy perspective on foods. Metabolic profiling helps identify the best ratio of proteins, carbohydrates and fats. A profile 1 does better on a high carb diet, a profile 2 does better on a higher protein diet and a profile 3 does better on a balanced diet. A profile 1 could use the "higher carb" ratio to justify a diet that is high in pasta, bread and sweets. This would meet the criteria of metabolic profiling but miss the goal of health.

A person following the glycemic index research would want to avoid the high glycemic index (GI) foods and consume more low glycemic foods. Consequently, he/she could "legally" support the health of a diet that includes chocolate fudge cake (GI of 38) instead of watermelon (GI of 72). Now all of us know fruit would be healthier than chocolate cake, but when it comes to blood insulin levels, that is not true. (See page 12 for more information on the Glycemic Index.)

Candida is the presence of a bad fungus in the body. Fungus grows in the presence of sugar. A diet to kill the presence of any fungus requires that all sugar be eliminated – in any form. With this factor, a client could choose to eat a bacon, egg and high protein diet without a balance of good carbohydrates (vegetables) and be "following" a Candida diet. Again, the rules would be followed, but health would not be the result.

Blood type cannot be ignored. We each have blood and each of us have one of the four blood types – O, A, B or AB. A blood type A can consume soy products, tamari and some cheeses. However, many of these foods can feed Candida, which is a common issue in blood type As.

The key is to use the focus of the research for each of these factors while not forgetting that health is the goal, not just the compliance to a program. No food plan should be the basis for approving unhealthy choices.

Common sense says we eat food. According to Webster's Unabridged 1953 dictionary, *food* is: "nutritive material absorbed into the body of an organism which serves for the purposes of:

- growth
- work
- repair or vital processes
- maintenance of vital processes."

To that end, all of the "no-no" foods still apply (white flour, white sugar, white rice, hydrogenated fats, preservatives, food dyes and other names on the label that you can't pronounce). When a food is allowed in any of our four factors that fits into the "no-no" list, it is by default omitted in the *Food Puzzle*.

Customization that is Easy to Use

You might be thinking that following any one of these eating plans would be too hard, so trying to combine *all four* would be impossible! It would be if you had to use four books and go back and forth between all four.

The beauty of the *Food Puzzle* is that it truly is easy to use. You simply build one layer upon the next layer. Here is how you can easily use the *Food Puzzle*, whether you are a health care provider working with clients, a mom or dad trying to get the family healthy or a single person wanting to lose weight.

Step 1: Eliminate the "No-No" Foods and Add the "Yes-Yes" Foods

The "no-no" list of foods has already been presented. Everyone knows the need to eliminate these foods, yet we often don't know where or how to start. When we started this process we were living on $850 per month. Our nutritionist told us to change our diet and eliminate these foods. Imagine my shock when I inventoried our pantry and found that over fifty percent of our food pantry contained those ingredients!!

My health was on the line, so I immediately cut out all of those foods and gave them away. I began the process of learning how to use whole grains, whole sweeteners and brown rice. Today, I find that whole foods taste better, are just as easy to prepare (once I learned how) and just as affordable.

The key was that I *learned* how to use them. If you are accustomed to using packaged foods, eating in fast food places and eating on the run, then eating foods that require some planning will require a paradigm shift and a time to learn how to do so. This step can and will take some time. The benefits are enormous and far outweigh the cost.

I highly recommend finding a good cookbook, an accountability partner and learning how to replace the "no-no" foods with the "yes-yes" foods. The "yes-yes" foods include:

- pure water
- fresh, organic (preferable) vegetables and fruits
- whole grains
- natural sweeteners (in moderation)
- organic meats, fish, eggs (if needed)
- fresh herbs

As important as supplements are, at Lifestyle for Health we focus on healthy foods and lots of pure water. Many health issues will disappear with just the subtraction of "no-no" foods and the addition of whole foods.

Step 2: Determine Your Metabolic Profile

The purpose of metabolic profiling is to determine your *ratio* of proteins, carbohydrates and fats. The chapter on metabolic profile goes into this subject in detail and it provides you with the metabolic profile questionnaire. Follow the directions and take the questionnaire. Be sure to also follow the scoring directions at the end of the survey.

Once you know your profile, review the information on your profile. This will give you your optimal food blend ratio and explain how to implement that ratio. Do not make it hard, keep it easy. The goal is to begin to eat *more* carbohydrates (from good sources) if you are a profile 1, *more* protein (from good sources) if you are a profile 2 and a *balance* of all three (from good sources) if you are a profile 3.

At this point you know the foods to avoid (white four, white sugar, white rice, hydrogenated fats and food dyes) and you know the ratio of your good foods. This is a key foundation for anybody. You are better off taking months to make this foundation solid, than to quickly try and implement the entire plan and only stick with it for a few weeks.

The goal in the *Food Puzzle* is to create an eating plan that you can live with the rest of your life. Learn to enjoy the process and take your time. It took you years to get to where you are and it will take time to reverse where you are. The good news is your body will manifest symptoms of health quickly when you begin to feed it healthy foods.

Step 3: Recognize and Eliminate High Glycemic Foods

An overview of the glycemic index (GI) is found later in this book. However, the index basically measures how much a food raises your blood sugar level and subsequent insulin response. The higher the number, the faster the rise in blood sugar and insulin levels. Consuming a diet high in foods that have a high GI contributes to high stress on the pancreas and is a leading contributor to hypoglycemia and diabetes.

In addition to raising blood sugar and insulin levels, a high GI food also lowers the body's ability to burn fat. High GI foods also increase appetite, affect mood swings and contribute to heart disease (the number one killer in the U.S.).

The glycemic index chapter will show you the glycemic score for commonly eaten foods to help you know foods to eliminate or use in moderation if you are dealing with hormonal imbalances, excess weight, diabetes or heart issues. As a basic rule, the more processing and refining that a food has gone through, the higher it's glycemic index will be.

Again, keep it simple. Do the basics first – avoid the "no-no, eat the "yes-yes" and eat the ratio that fits your profile. Now you can begin to avoid the high glycemic foods. As you read the list, you will note that rice cakes have a high GI score. Rice cakes are not a good snack, although they can be made more balanced by adding almond butter. The key is that rice cakes, although low in fat, are high on the GI scale; this is a good example of what happens to a food (brown rice) when it is highly processed. The glycemic index of rice cakes is almost twice that of brown rice.

You will also notice that potatoes are high glycemic foods, with baked potatoes being among the highest. The key is to realize that baked potatoes are high on the scale and should be consumed in moderation. If you want to lose weight, then they are not your *best* choice. However, as you eliminate the "no-no" foods you will be eliminating many high GI foods. Don't get legalistic, a baked potato on occasion will not hurt you. However, potatoes at every meal would not be good.

In our glycemic list you will note that we have left out many packaged and processed foods. That is because we don't include them in our "optimal food" list, and so even with a low glycemic score, we would not eat them.

Step 4: Test for Candida

Candida and fungal imbalances are estimated to impact one in three Americans. I find it is very common among blood type As. The Candida questionnaire is a simple, self-scoring test that allows you to identify the possible presence of Candida. I have never found a person to be harmed by doing a Candida cleanse or by following a Candida diet. If you have any questions regarding a cleanse, I recommend you work with your health care provider or a LFH Coach.

In your implementation process, I recommend you carefully plan when you will do a Candida cleanse/diet. I personally do one once a year, usually after the holidays. Do not plan to start a cleanse during Christmas or some other key holiday. Do not plan to do a cleanse during a vacation or during a holiday.

Pick your time wisely and then plan how you will handle any difficult times such as social occasions. Most cleanses need to last at least one month. The key during a Candida cleanse is to stop feeding the fungus and use the cleansing products to kill the existing fungus. The closer you follow the diet the shorter the cleanse time will need to be. The Candida chapter will give you additional insight in implementing this part of the *Food Puzzle*.

If your score was low on the Candida Questionnaire, skip that section and go to the blood type section.

Step 5: Learn About Your Blood Type

The blood type diet has been excellently covered by Dr. Peter J. D'Adamo in his informative books *Eat Right for Your Blood Type* and *Live Right for Your Type*. He has excellent research and I highly recommend both books.

The problem I found in using blood types alone, is that what we have already covered is overlooked. For example, I am a blood type A and should do well on a mostly vegetarian diet. However, I am also a profile 2, which calls for higher protein and I do not produce purine (see the metabolic profile chapter). When I followed either the blood type or the metabolic profile plans exclusively I found I lacked energy and gained weight. When I combined them into the *Food Puzzle*, I did much better.

I also believe that unclean meat and fish should be avoided. They are scavengers and a leading contributor to parasites. These foods have been eliminated from our eating guidelines. (For a list of unclean meats and fish, see the Blood Type Overview.)

The other key to the blood type information is the correlation to exercise, disease, emotional issues and recommended supplements. This section was completely developed based on my experience with thousands of clients. This section can be invaluable to practitioners when dealing with health issues in clients with different blood types.

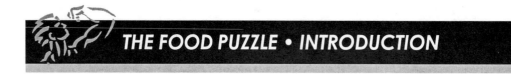

Step 6: Keep it Simple
If/When you get confused, go back to the basics ...
- Avoid the "no-no" foods
- Eat the "yes-yes" foods
- Drink pure water
- Relax!

Any food eaten under stress – emotional or physical – causes poor digestion. I found this beautifully noted by one of our clients. She had really been following her *Food Puzzle* and was feeling quite good. She took a cruise and enjoyed a few "no-no" foods, although she was selective in her choices and did not binge at every meal. She was relaxed and did great. She returned home and thought she no longer needed to follow the *Food Puzzle*. She ate a donut at church and immediately felt lousy, was tired and experienced reactions for a day or two.

What was the difference? Stress. On the cruise she was relaxed and so was her digestion. At home, she was back into the stress of her daily routine. The higher the stress, the closer you need to follow the *Food Puzzle*. The less the stress the more casual you can be.

If you become obsessive over your eating plan, then you will miss many of the benefits of eating well. The key is to do as much as you can without stressing over it. I often find people do better by going slower and staying relaxed than going full force ahead and getting stressed. If you tend to stress, then I highly recommend the use of a flower essence called Rock Water. Rock Water helps people who tend to be perfectionistic and hard on themselves. Flower therapies can be discussed with your health care provider or with a LFH Coach.

Step 7: Work With a Health Care Coach
My health has come a long way since 1989 when I attempted suicide, had a significant weight problem and experienced an emotional breakdown. I could never have made the changes I made without the knowledge, accountability and structure provided by my nutritionist.

We see this all the time at Lifestyle for Health. The clients who are accountable to a coach and are willing to make changes one step at a time are the ones that see the most significant changes and changes that last. I have watched people do well for a short period of time because they are on a "quick-fix" plan to lose weight without consideration of their overall health. They lose their weight, then gain more back and quickly join the vast number of American weight loss yo-yo'ers. Don't do that to yourself! You deserve better.

Take the time to find a practitioner who has good fruit – who is healthy or in the process of getting healthier. If they have the fruit of health in their life, then they have something to offer you. A good health care provider is a valuable mentor that can help you avoid pitfalls, keep costs down and keep you motivated when you feel like quitting. This kind of service is invaluable!

However, a practitioner who has not developed health in his/her own life and is only focused on selling you products can be a source of much frustration. Take the time to interview. Check out references. Remember, you pay the bill, you are the boss – so you can hire who you want. Hire the best you can and then listen to what they say.

Learn to ask good questions (wisdom is the ability to know what question to ask and of whom to ask it). Make good use of your time with your practitioner. Be accountable – be willing to make the changes they recommend. Doing what you have always done will get you what you have. To get something different you must do something different. The key is to know what to do differently.

The *Food Puzzle* is designed with you in mind. *Combine it with the skill of a competent health care provider and your commitment to optimal health and you have a winning combination each and every time!*

Many good health care providers exist around the country. Lifestyle for Health is committed to developing proven strategies that can be used by practitioners beyond our office. If you are looking for a health care provider, we invite you to check out LFH. If you have a practitioner and you have found the *Food Puzzle* to be of help, share the news with him/her. Any practitioner can use the *Food Puzzle* in his/her practice. If you are a practitioner and are interested in the LFH Coaching Program, give us a call. Our number can be found on the order form at the back of the book.

May God bless you as you unravel the puzzle of what to eat. Make it an adventure and have fun along the away. Learn to eat what your body was designed to eat, and you will begin to experience renewed health. Remember, health is not the destination; it is simply the vehicle that allows you to live out your God-given potential and enjoy life to the fullest.

METABOLIC PROFILING

What Is Metabolic Profiling?

Metabolic Profiling is a system of interpreting and understanding body language to determine an individual's genetically-based nutritional requirements. In the 1980s Dr. William D. Kelley developed a computerized system of metabolic profiling that was based on the genetic influence on the autonomic nervous system. More than 10,000 patients were enlisted into the program, which has provided one of the largest collections of data ever compiled on metabolic profiling and individualized nutrition.

Members of Kelley's research team later expanded this computerized analysis to look beyond the autonomic influence and into the interrelationship of the body's three main systems responsible for the creation, maintenance and control of energy. These three systems are the autonomic nervous system, the oxidative system and the endocrine system

The autonomic system controls all involuntary activity in the body, such as digestion, elimination, heart beat and immune activity. It is comprised of two divisions: sympathetic (process of fight/flight and adrenal stress) and parasympathetic (process of needing rest/relaxation and adrenal fatigue). The oxidative system is concerned with the rate at which nutrients are converted to energy in the cells through a process called oxidation. The endocrine system exerts its influence on cellular metabolism through the secretion of hormones, which are essential for the regulation of all activities in the body.

Genetically, each person has inherited various strengths and weaknesses in each of these systems. Some people are more strongly influenced by the sympathetic part of the autonomic nervous system. Others are influenced more strongly by the parasympathetic system. Some people are fast oxidizers, others tend to be slow oxidizers. Those variances provide the basis for all of our physiological, psychological and diet-related characteristics.

For example, sympathetic types tend to have high energy and excellent concentration, yet tend to also have weak digestion and dry skin. Slow oxidizers tend to burn their foods too slowly and can thus have poor appetites. Each individual nutrient:
- can have a more pronounced influence on either the parasympathetic or sympathetic system
- can affect either fast or slow oxidation OR
- can trigger a particular endocrine gland

What Is Your Metabolic Profile?

A key to determining a well-balanced diet for you is to first identify your metabolic profile. Once you know your profile, you can eat the right ratio of nutrients to take advantage of your strengths while supporting your metabolic weaknesses. This helps to balance the body's energy-producing systems, thus promoting optimal cellular balance – in other words promoting homeostasis or optimal health.

Research has now provided the most scientifically based system of metabolic profiling yet available. The result of an evolutionary process, the research spanned some 25 years and involved the synthesis of extensive empirical research and clinical experiences of approximately 30,000 subjects. In 1996 the first self-scoring metabolic profiling survey was developed from this enormous database and was subsequently licensed to Mannatech, Inc. Their pioneering metabolic profiling survey is included here by their permission.

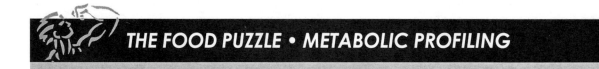

Metabolic Profile Survey and Product Selection Guide

Instructions:
- Place a check (✓) in the square to the left of each choice that best applies to you.
- Make only one selection per category.
- If no choice applies to you, leave that category unchecked.
- **Important:** The choices as written may not describe you exactly. So, it is very important that you choose an answer that best describes your tendencies. The answer doesn't need to be a perfect description, just an indication of your trend.
- Consider letting a close friend or family member check your answers for accuracy.
- Be as honest and accurate as you can. After all, you want to be sure to obtain the right product for your kind of metabolism.
- Some choices in some columns are purposefully left blank.

CHARACTERISTIC	☑ COLUMN 1	☑ COLUMN 2	☑ COLUMN 3
Aging	☐ Look older than others my age	☑ Look younger than others my age	☐
Aloofness	☑ Cool, distant, aloof, loner, slow to make friends, hard to get to know	☐ Warm, open, expressive, easily make friends, approachable	☐
Appetite	☐ Weak, lacking, diminished	☐ Strong, excessive, enhanced	☑ Average appetite
Chest Pressure	☐	☐ Tend to get	☐
Climate	☑ Love warm, hot weather	☐ Do well in cold, poor in hot	☑ Doesn't matter
Cold Sores and/or Fever Blisters	☐	☐ Tend to get	☐
Coughing	☐	☐ Tend to cough most every day	☐
Cracking Skin (any weather)	☐	☐ Tend to get	☐
Dandruff	☐	☐ Tend to get	☐
Desserts	☐ Love sweets, need something sweet with meal to feel satisfied or salty (like cheese, chips or popcorn) for snacks after meals	☐ Don't really care for sweet desserts, but like something fatty	☑ Can take them or leave them
Digestion	☐ Poor, weak, slow	☐ Good, strong, rapid	☑ Average digestion
Eating Before Bed	☐ Usually worsens sleep, especially if heavy food	☐ Usually improves sleep	☑ Doesn't matter, but heavy snacks
Eating Habits	☐ Eat to live - unconcerned with food and eating	☐ Live to eat - need to eat often to feel good, be at best	☑ Average eating habits and need for food, meal times, etc.
Emotional Expression	☐ Hard to express feelings, not naturally demonstrative	☑ Easily express feelings	☐
Emotions	☑ Beneath surface, under control, non-emotional type, tend to hold feelings inside	☐ Wear heart on sleeve, others always know how I feel	☐
Eye Moisture	☑ Tend toward dry eyes	☐ Tend toward moist or tearing eyes	☐
Facial Coloring	☑ Tend toward pale, chalky	☐ Tend toward ruddy, rosy, flushed	☐
Facial Complexion	☐ Tend toward dull, unclear	☑ Tend toward bright, clear	☐

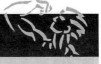

CHARACTERISTIC	✔ COLUMN 1	✔ COLUMN 2	✔ COLUMN 3
Fatty Food (if you like or dislike, not what you think is good for you)	☐ Don't care for it	☐ Love it, crave it, would like it often	☑ Take it or leave it
Fatty Food Reaction	☐ Decreases energy and well-being	☐ Increased well-being	☑ Average reaction
Fingernails	☑ Tend to be thick, hard, strong	☐ Tend to be thin, soft, weak	☐
4 Hours Without Eating	☐ Doesn't bother	☐ Makes irritable, jittery, weak famished or depressed	☑ Feel normal hunger
Gooseflesh	☑ Tend to form easily	☐	☐
Gum Bleeding	☐	☐ Tend to get after brushing	☐
Gum Color	☑ Light, pale	☐ Dark, pink, red	☐
Hunger Feelings	☐ Rarely get, passes quickly, can go long periods w/o eating easily	☑ Often hungry, need to eat regularly and often	☐ When late for meals only, not between meals usually
Insect Bite	☑ Weak reaction, disappears fast	☐ Strong, lasting reaction	☐
Itching Eyes	☐	☐ Tend to get	☐ Average reaction
Juice or Water Fasting	☐ Can handle very well, feels good	☑ Fasting makes me feel awful	☐ React O.K., can fast if necessary
Meal Portions	☐ Prefer small	☐ Prefer large, or if not large, need it often	☑ Average
Orange Juice Alone	☐ Energizes, satisfies me	☐ Can make me light-headed, hungry, jittery, shaky, or nauseated	☑ No ill effects
Potatoes	☑ Not real fond of them	☐ Could eat them almost everyday, love them	☐ Take them or leave them
Red Meat, like a steak or roast beef meal	☐ Decreases energy and well-being	☐ Increases energy and well-being	☑ Average reaction
Saliva Amount	☐ Tend toward dry mouth	☑ Excessive saliva	☐
Saliva Texture	☐ Tends to be thick, ropy	☑ Tends to be thin, watery	☐
Salty Foods	☐ Foods often taste too salty	☐ Really love or crave salt on foods	☑ Average like for
Skin Healing	☐ Cuts heal slowly	☐ Cuts heal quickly	☑ Average healing time
Skin Moisture	☑ Tend toward dry skin	☐ Tend toward oily/moist skin	☐ Average skin moisture
Skipping Meals	☐ Can skip with no ill effects	☑ Must eat regularly (or often)	☐ Can get by w/o eating but really feel best eating 3 meals per day
Snacking	☐ Rarely or never want snacks	☑ Want to eat between meals	☐
Sneezing (any time)	☐	☐ Tend to sneeze every day	☐
Sour Foods (vinegar, pickles, lemons, sauerkraut or yogurt)	☐ Don't care for, want or crave	☐ Really like	☑ Sometimes like
Sweets	☐ Can do fairly well on	☐ Don't do well on, sweet foods can seem too sweet	☑ No noticeable bad effect
Vegetarian Meals	☑ Is satisfying	☐ Not satisfying, or bad result, become hungry soon after or feel unsatisfied	☐ O.K., but not really satisfying

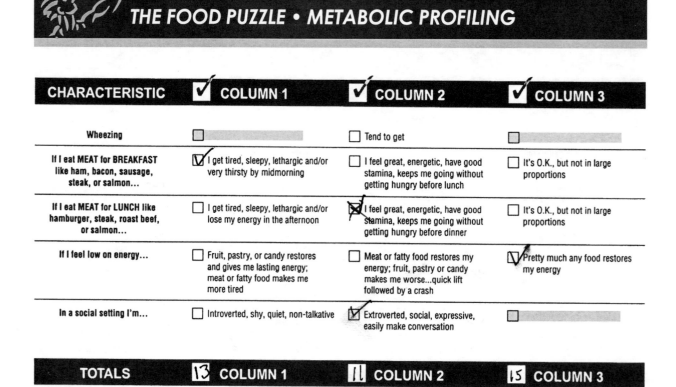

CHARACTERISTIC	☑ COLUMN 1	☑ COLUMN 2	☑ COLUMN 3
Wheezing	☐	☐ Tend to get	☐
If I eat MEAT for BREAKFAST like ham, bacon, sausage, steak, or salmon...	☑ I get tired, sleepy, lethargic and/or very thirsty by midmorning	☐ I feel great, energetic, have good stamina, keeps me going without getting hungry before lunch	☐ It's O.K., but not in large proportions
If I eat MEAT for LUNCH like hamburger, steak, roast beef, or salmon...	☐ I get tired, sleepy, lethargic and/or lose my energy in the afternoon	☑ I feel great, energetic, have good stamina, keeps me going without getting hungry before dinner	☐ It's O.K., but not in large proportions
If I feel low on energy...	☐ Fruit, pastry, or candy restores and gives me lasting energy; meat or fatty food makes me more tired	☐ Meat or fatty food restores my energy; fruit, pastry or candy makes me worse...quick lift followed by a crash	☑ Pretty much any food restores my energy
In a social setting I'm...	☐ Introverted, shy, quiet, non-talkative	☑ Extroverted, social, expressive, easily make conversation	☐
TOTALS	13 COLUMN 1	11 COLUMN 2	15 COLUMN 3

Steps for Product Selection:

Great. That way easy, right? Now, on to finding out which product to order... Just follow these steps:

1. Add up the total choices made in each column and enter your total score in the space provided at the end of each column.
2. If your highest score in one column is 5 points or more higher than both of the other two columns, and...

   if you made the most choices in column 1, Profile #1 is the product for you.

   ...if you made the most choices in column 2, Profile #2 is the product for you.

   ...if you made the most choices in column 3, Profile #3 is the product for you.

   If the column with your highest score is not 5 points or higher than both of the other two columns, find your results below:
3. If column 1 and column 2 are tied or have less than 5 points difference, Profile #3 is for you.
4. If column 1 and column 3 are tied or have less than 5 points difference, Profile #1 is for you.
5. If column 2 and column 3 are tied or have less than 5 points difference, Profile #2 is for you.
6. If all three columns are tied or have scores with 5 points or less difference (e.g. 13, 18, 16), Profile #3 is the product for you.

It's quite possible that due to various factors such as time, age, stress and activity levels, etc., your nutritional needs could change. Whenever you feel that a change may have taken place, answer the questions above and re-do the steps for product selection. Good luck and enjoy.

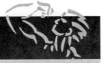

The Three Metabolic Profiles

Profile 1 • Slow Burner

Daily Intake

Protein
- 20% daily intake
- 4 – 6 ounces low-fat protein
- 2 nonfat dairy servings, if tolerated

Carbohydrates
- 70% daily intake
- 4+ servings of vegetables
- 4+ servings of complex carbohydrates
- 2 – 4 servings of fruit

Fats
- 10% daily intake
- 1 tablespoon of essential fatty acids (EFAs) and healthy fats
- 1 serving of oils, nuts, nut butters

Water
- 8 – 10 8-ounce glasses of water

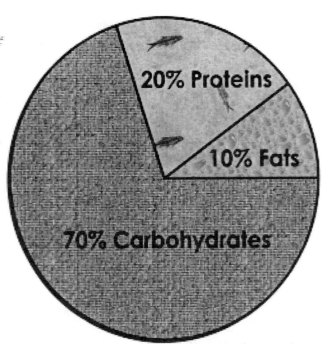

Keys ... primarily vegetarian, high carbohydrate concentration

Profile 1

People who score high as a profile 1 burn their food slowly. They may tend toward high blood sugar or diabetic problems. They may notice they have a poor appetite and dislike protein-rich foods. They often have an inefficient glandular system and show problems with the thyroid and/or adrenal glands. They may also experience fatigue, exhaustion, depression and sense of being cold.

This profile can be a problem for those having blood type O. Profile 1 is more vegetarian and blood type O does better on protein, especially some red meat. A profile 1, blood type O requires a little more fine-tuning then those of the other blood types. If you are such a person, you might really benefit from working with a LFH Coach.

Profile 2 • Fast Burner

Daily Intake

Protein
- 45 – 50% daily intake
- 6 – 8 ounces low-fat protein
- 2 higher fat dairy servings, if tolerated

Carbohydrates
- 30 – 35% daily intake
- 4+ servings of vegetables
- 2+ servings of complex carbohydrates
- 1 – 2 servings of fruit

Fats
- 20% daily intake
- 2 tablespoons of EFAs
- 2 – 4 servings of oils, nuts, nut butters

Water
- 8 – 10 8-ounce glasses of water

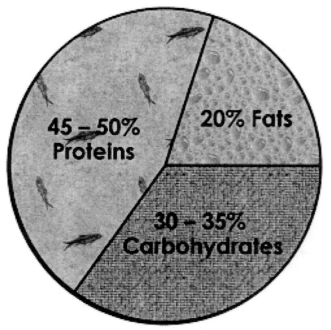

Keys ... higher protein diet

Profile 2

People who score as a profile 2 need a higher level of protein as they ten to burn their food too quickly. They may often feel hyped up, nervous and/or easily stressed. They also may have low blood sugar and are often diagnosed as hypoglycemic. They may show wider mood swings, especially when they go too long without eating. They usually have stronger appetites than the profile 1. Children or adults with Attention Deficit Disorder (ADD) or Attention Deficit Hyperactivity Disorder (ADHD) are often profile 2. Excessive carbohydrates will cause a quick rush of energy and then a crash, along with excess weight.

The challenge in this group is for those who are profile 2 and blood type A. Again, the profile 2 requires higher levels of protein (including purine-rich foods†), while the blood type A is more vegetarian. Unlike the other profiles, the profile 2 does not make purines in the body, these amino acids must come from the diet. Profile 2, blood type A is sensitive and requires more sensitive balancing of protein, often requiring additional enzyme support to assimilate the protein. If you have questions on this area, please call the LFH office and schedule a time with a Coach.

†Purine is a special class of proteins, called nucleoproteins, that are excellent sources of energy for fast burners, but not slow burners. Slow burners produce this energy in their cells, whereas fast burners do not.
- Purine-rich fish sources includes caviar, herring anchovies
- Purine-rich meat sources includes beef, organ meats, veal, wild game

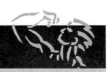
Profile 3 • Balanced Burner

Daily Intake

Protein
- 40 – 45% daily requirement
- 4 – 6 ounces low-fat protein
- 2 dairy servings if tolerated

Carbohydrates
- 50 – 55% daily requirement
- 4+ servings of vegetables
- 4+ servings of complex carbohydrates (whole grains)
- 1 – 4 servings of fruit

Fats
- 10 – 15% daily requirement
- 1 – 2 tablespoons of EFAs
- 2 – 4 servings of oils, nuts, nut butters

Water
- 8 – 10 8-ounce glasses of water

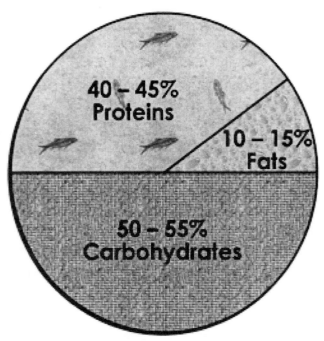

Keys ... balanced fuel blend

Profile 3

People who score high as a profile 3 do not have the sensitivity to nutrient balancing as the other two profiles do. This group can easily blend the nutrients according to the above ratio.

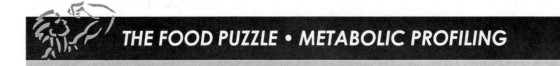
Notes on Metabolic Profiling

GLYCEMIC INDEX

What Is the Glycemic Index?

The glycemic index (GI) is a clinical rating of the impact of a food on the insulin of the body. The index was first developed in 1981 by a team of scientists. Dr. David Jenkins, a professor of nutrition at the University of Toronto, Canada helped lead this team. Their research was focused on which foods were best for diabetics.

The carbohydrate exchange program that was being used by diabetics was confusing and complicated. Jenkins approach went against the prevailing belief that all carbohydrates impacted the body the same. He believed and studied the diverse impact of different carbohydrates on real people.

The Glycemic Research Institute (GRI) is a non-profit, non-partisan organization based in Washington D.C. that conducts clinical analytic studies of the impact of foods, drinks, packaged foods, nutrients and nutraceuticals. The Institute has compiled and recorded the GI for thousands of foods and food products. A non-partisan organization, the Institute tests foods and products to determine their GI.

Foods that elicit a low glycemic response are licensed to use the Seal of Approval from the Glycemic Research Institute, which can be displayed on the label. It is an Food and Drug Administration (FDA) violation to print incorrect information, such as stating a product is "low glycemic" on a label, if it is not. The GRI Seal of Approval is provided pro-bono to manufacturers whose products qualify.

Several factors impact the GI. Those factors include:

- Cooking and Processing.
  Cooking and processing increases the GI of a food as it increases the amount of gelatinized starch in the food. Example: rice cakes have a higher GI than plain, cooked rice.
- Form of Food.
  Food in its natural form has a lower GI. Example: whole wheat has a lower GI than wheat bread (not 100% whole), which in turn is lower than refined white bread.
- Fiber.
  Fiber content slows down the digestion of a food and thereby lowers that food's GI. Example: higher fiber fruits (i.e., apples) have a lower GI.
- Sugar.
  The type of sugar makes a difference. Example: fruit-based sugar (fructose) breaks down slowly, so most fruits have a low GI.

Why is the Glycemic Index Important?

Glucose is given a relative value of 100 in the glycemic table and all other foods and substances are given scores based on that basis. The higher the glycemic index of a food the faster the hit of glucose in the body. The lower the glycemic index of a food the slower the release of glucose into the blood stream. Why is that important? *The rate at which your blood sugar rises after eating is crucial in balancing weight!* High levels of glucose in the blood cause the release of insulin. Insulin is responsible for causing the storage of excess glucose in the form of fat.

Eating foods with high glycemic ratings can cause the following problems:

- increased appetite

- impact mood swings
- increased fat storage (obesity and/or weight gain)
- increase in adipose (fat) tissue on the body
- excess insulin in the blood stream
- increased risk of Type II (adult-onset) diabetes
- increased risk of reactive hypoglycemia
- increased risk of heart disease
- increased triglyceride production

Since the glycemic index measures the impact of a food on blood sugar, there is no GI for meat, fish or fowl. Therefore, they are not found in any GI table, unless the indication is "none." Dairy products will be listed if they contain lactose, which is a dairy sugar. All other foods contain some type of carbohydrate and have a GI score.

Many people mistakenly believe that the GI is a sugar rating alone. However, this is not true. Some of the highest GI foods are starchy, processed foods such as refined bread, breakfast cereals and potato products.

Research continues to point to low-fat, high glycemic diets as a main contributor to weight gain in the U.S. The U.S. leads in the production of "low-fat" foods and also, according to the World Health Organization, leads the world in obesity. "Low-fat" is not the answer to being low fat!

Low glycemic foods include:

- whole grains
- whole fruits
- whole beans
- whole vegetables
- yogurt
- nuts

High glycemic foods include:

- carrot, beet and celery juices
- processed grains and products using refined flour
- white rice
- potatoes, French fries
- processed cereals, crackers, canned/packaged pastas, chips, pretzels, popcorn
- ice cream
- refined sugar and products using refined sugar
- drinks/foods made with: maltodextrins, glucose polymers, corn syrup, dextrins, high fructose corn syrup
- non-dairy whipped toppings (lite or regular)
- instant pudding mixes
- sweetened condensed milk
- pizza
- jelly beans, Life Savers, most candy bars

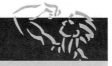

A table of commonly eaten foods and their GI can be found at the end of this section. *The Food Puzzle* indicates high GI foods for you. Eliminating those foods will help you with weight loss and blood sugar balancing. The index at the end of this section is to simply help you recognize the GI index of commonly eaten foods.

How Does Insulin Impact the Picture?

We know that food breaks down to glucose, which is the basis of blood sugar. So how does insulin fit into the picture?

Insulin was discovered in 1921. It is manufactured and secreted by the pancreas, which stores about 200 units of insulin. The average person secretes about 25 – 30 units per day. Insulin acts like a broom, sweeping glucose, amino acids and free fatty acids into cells to be stored as fat and glycogen by the liver for future use. In a healthy person, glucose and insulin levels have little fluctuation. However, a person cannot live without insulin.

Glucagon, also made by the pancreas, prevents blood sugar from falling too low. The main role of this hormone is to prevent hypoglycemia or low blood sugar. Glucagon secretion is stimulated by hypoglycemia, fasting and the ingestion of protein-rich meals.

Glucose is the major stimulus for insulin secretion. Other sugars (i.e., fructose, lactose) can cause a release of insulin only in the presence of previously elevated blood sugar. This means that overweight people can have more insulin production and even get to the point of "insulin resistance," making it even harder to lose weight.

"Insulin resistance" is a condition of decreased responsiveness to insulin where fat, liver and muscle cells have become insensitive to normal levels of circulating insulin. In an "insulin resistant" individual, more insulin is required to lower blood sugar (glucose). The most common results of being "insulin resistant" are excess weight, obesity and Type II diabetes.

"Insulin resistance" can also impact blood cholesterol levels and corresponding imbalances in adrenaline. That is why, at LFH, we check the status of the adrenals. If the adrenals are stressed it is very common to see elevated levels of insulin, cholesterol and other hormones (i.e. cortisol and estrogen).

How can "insulin resistance" be reduced? Following a low-glycemic diet and monitoring adrenal stress can greatly help! Exercise also helps this process. Research bears out these statements.

1. Dr. Wolever, in 1992, studied the benefits of a low-glycemic index diet on over-weight, non-insulin-dependent diabetics. They found a 7% drop in cholesterol after only six weeks.
2. Dr. Jenkins, in 1987, studied a low-glycemic diet on normal males. After two weeks the men's cholesterol dropped an average of 15% and insulin secretion dropped 32%.

Are All Sweeteners the Same?

Many sweeteners are on the market. My personal belief is that whole, natural sweeteners (even if they are higher GI) combined with whole grain flours make for a better "treat" than a product made from refined sugars and refined flours. It is not what you consume 5% of the time, it is what you consume 95% of the time that makes the difference. For that "occasional treat," learn to make wholesome desserts (see a good cookbook such as the *Lifestyle for Health Cookbook*) or purchase products made

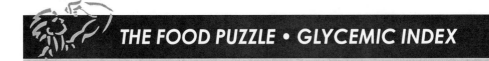

from whole foods. Treats eaten as dessert with a balanced meal are "easier" on the system than those eaten on an empty stomach with no "real food" to balance out the sudden increase in sugars.

The following is a review of sweeteners and how they fit into the GI scale.

Sugar	Comments
Low Glycemic	
Fructose	low GI (23) 1½ times sweeter than sugar natural fruit sugar
Trutina Dulcem	low GI (score not available) 15 times sweeter than sugar or fructose 1 teaspoon of Trutina is equal to 15 teaspoons of sugar
Medium Glycemic	
Sucrose	medium GI (65) common table sugar, made up of glucose and fructose. Americans consume 65 pounds per year. Americans consume 150 pounds of all *refined* sugars per year.
FruitSource	medium GI (score not available) A dried blend of grape juice concentrate and whole rice syrup. The GI is higher than that of sucrose.
High Glycemic	
Honey	high GI
Barley malt	high GI
Date sugar	high GI
Brown sugar	high GI Similar to sucrose, with the addition of some molasses
Raw sugar	high GI 96% sucrose and 4% molasses
Turbinado sugar	high GI 95% sucrose and 55% molasses
Corn syrup	high GI

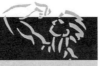
| High fructose corn syrup | high GI Not the same as fructose, prepared from corn syrup and glucose |

High fructose
corn syrup — high GI
Not the same as fructose, prepared from corn syrup and glucose

Maple syrup — high GI

Molasses — high GI
High mineral content does help.

Sucanat — high GI

Very High Glycemic
Maltodextrins — very high GI

Glucose Polymers — very high GI

Other
Mannitol — Natural sweetener found in asparagus, pineapples, olives and seaweed. Causes less sugar rise than sucrose and glucose. Poor absorption by the intestine results in osmotic diarrhea. High intake can act as a laxative and worsen kidney disease.

Sorbitol — Naturally occurring sugar alcohol, made from glucose.
Large intake (50g.) can cause diarrhea. It cannot leak out of cells and can gradually accumulate, leading to tissue damage and osmotic imbalances.

Xylitol — Made from bark sugar found in fruits and vegetables. Commercially source is birch bark. No effect on blood sugar. Can cause diarrhea,. Animals consuming xylitol for long periods have developed bladder and adrenal tumors.

Maltitol — Low GI. Made by hydrogenation of maltose.

Stevia — Low GI. Sweet herb, not recognized as a legal sugar in the U.S. (as of 2/99) Certain stevia products contain high glycemic maltodextrins. Check label for contents.

Agave Syrup — Low GI. Made from Agave plant. Known effects of the Agave plant include disintegration of red blood cells, depression of the central nervous system and cellular damage.

Summary

Understanding the GI of foods is essential in controlling overproduction of insulin, developing "insulin resistance" and the stimulation of adipose (fat) tissue. Eating foods with a high GI increases appetite and weight. By reducing the intake of high GI foods, a person can lower the risk of diabetes, heart disease, and obesity, while increasing energy and sense of well being.

Check out the following tables to determine high GI foods you may be eating. These foods will be highlighted in your "beneficial" and "neutral" lists later in the *Food Puzzle*. We have not included most processed, packaged or "junk foods" on this list as they tend to be high on the glycemic scale, have minimal nutritional value and are not part of the Lifestyle for Health optimal eating plan! Scores over 70 are considered High and scores under 50 are considered Low.

Beans

Soy beans, boiled, ½ cup	18
Kidney beans, red, boiled, ½ cup	27
Black beans, boiled, ¾ cup	30
Kidney beans, red, canned, ½ cup	30
Lentils, green and brown, boiled, ½ cup	30
Butter beans, boiled, ½ cup	31
Cannellini beans, ½ cup	31
Lima beans, baby, frozen, ½ cup	32
Split peas, yellow, boiled, ½ cup	32
Chickpeas, (garbanzo beans), boiled, ½ cup	33
Garbanzo beans, boiled, ½ cup	33
Mung beans, boiled, ½ cup	38
Navy beans, boiled, ½ cup	38
Pinto beans, soaked, boiled, ½ cup	39
Blackeyed peas, canned, ½ cup	42
Chickpeas (garbanzo beans), canned, ½ cup	42
Garbanzo beans, canned, ½ cup	42
Peas, dried, boiled, ½ cup	45
Baked beans, ½ cup	48
Peas, green, fresh, frozen, boiled, ½ cup	48
Broad beans, canned, ½ cup	79
Fava beans, frozen, boiled, ½ cup	79
Lentils, red, boiled, ½ cup	26

Breads

100% stone ground whole wheat, 1 slice	53
American rye, 1	68
Bread stuffing from mix, 2 oz.	74
Dark rye, black bread, 1 slice	76
French baguette, 1 oz.	95
Gluten-free bread, 1 slice	90
Kaiser roll, 1	73

Breads, continued

Melba toast, 6 pieces	70
Pita bread, whole wheat, 6½ inch loaf	57
Pumpernickel, whole grain,1 slice	51
Rye bread, 1 slice	65
Sourdough, 1 slice	52
White, 1 slice	70
Whole wheat, 1 slice	69

Dairy/Non-Dairy

Ice cream, 10% fat, vanilla, ½ cup	61
Ice milk, vanilla, ½ cup	50
Milk, skim, 1 cup	32
Milk, whole, 1 cup	27
Soy milk, 1 cup	31
Tofu, frozen dessert, low fat, ½ cup	115
Yogurt, non-fat, fruit flavored with sugar, 8 oz.	33
Yogurt, non-fat, plain, no sugar	14

Fruit

Apple juice, unsweetened, 1 cup, 8 oz	40
Apple, 1 medium, 5 oz.	38
Apple, dried, 1 oz.	29
Apricot jam, no added sugar, 1 tablespoon	55
Apricots, dried, 1 oz.	31
Apricots, fresh, 3 medium, 3.3 oz	57
Banana, raw, 1 medium, 5 oz.	55
Cherries, 10 large, 3 oz.	22
Cranberry juice cocktail, 8 oz	52
Dates, dried, 5, 1.4 oz	103
Fruit cocktail, canned in natural juice, ½ cup	55
Grapefruit juice, unsweetened, 1 cup	48
Grapefruit, raw, ½ medium	25
Grapes, green, 1 cup	46
Kiwi, 1 medium, raw, peeled	52
Mango, 1 small	55
Marmalade	48
Orange juice, 1 cup	46
Orange, navel, 1 medium	44
Papaya, ½ medium	58
Peach, canned, light syrup, ½ cup	52
Peach, canned, natural juice, ½ cup	30
Peach, fresh, 1 medium	30
Peach, heavy syrup, ½ cup	58

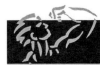

Fruit, continued

Pear, canned in pear juice, ½ cup	44
Pear, fresh, 1 medium	38
Pineapple juice, unsweetened, canned, 8 oz.	46
Pineapple, fresh, 2 slices, 4 oz.	66
Plums, 1 medium	39
Prunes, pitted	29
Raisins, ¼ cup	64
Strawberry jam, 1 tablespoon	51
Watermelon, 1 cup	72

Grains

Barley, pearled, boiled, ½ cup	25
Brown rice, 1 cup	55
Bulgur, cooked, ½ cup	48
Corn, canned, drained, ½ cup	69
Cornmeal, whole grain, cooked ⅓ cup	68
Couscous, cooked, ½ cup	65
Jasmine rice, 1 cup	109
Oat bran, 1 tablespoon	55
Rice bran, 1 tablespoon	19
Rice cakes, 3 cakes	82
Rice, basmati, white, boiled, 1 cup	58
Rice, brown, 1 cup	55
Rice, instant, white, cooked, 1 cup	56
Rice, long grain, white, 1 cup	56
Rice, short grain, white, 1 cup	72

Snacks

Corn chips, 1 oz	72
Potato chips, 14 pieces	54
Premium saltine crackers, 8 crackers	74
Pretzels, 1 oz.	83
Soft drink, 1 can	63
Vanilla wafers, 7 cookies	77
Water crackers, 3 king size crackers	78

Sweeteners

Honey, 1 tablespoon	61
Sucrose, table sugar, 1 tablespoon	65

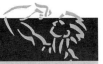

Vegetables

Artichokes, cooked, ½ cup	0 – 15
Asparagus, cooked, ½ cup	0 – 15
Beans, green, ½ cup	0 – 15
Beets, canned, drained, ½ cup	64
Bell peppers, raw, ½ cup	0 – 15
Broccoli, raw or steamed, ½ cup	0 – 15
Brussels sprouts, raw or steamed, ½ cup	0 – 15
Cabbage, shredded, ½ cup	0 – 15
Carrots, peeled, boiled, ½ cup	49
Cauliflower, raw or steamed, ½ cup	0 – 15
Celery, raw, ½ cup	0 – 15
Cucumbers, raw, ½ cup	0 – 15
Eggplant, cooked, ½ cup	0 – 15
French fries, 4.3 oz.	75
Lettuce, raw, 1 cup	0 – 15
Mushrooms, cooked, ½ cup	0 – 15
Okra, cooked, ½ cup	0 – 15
Onions, raw or cooked, ½ cup	0 – 15
Parsnips, boiled, ½ cup	95
Potatoes, baked in oven, 1 medium	93
Potatoes, mashed, ½ cup	91
Potatoes, new, unpeeled, boiled, 4 medium	78
Potatoes, red-skinned, peeled, boiled, 1 medium	88
Potatoes, white skin, baked, 1 medium	85
Potatoes, white skin, peeled, boiled, 1 medium	63
Potatoes, white skin, peeled, mashed, ½ cup	70
Pumpkin, peeled, boiled, mashed, ½ cup	75
Radishes, raw, ½ cup	0 – 15
Spinach, cooked, ½ cup	0 – 15
Spinach, raw, 1 cup	0 – 15
Squash, cooked, ½ cup	0 – 15
Sweet potato, peeled, boiled, mashed, ½ cup	54
Turnip green, raw, 1 cup	0 – 15
Zucchini, cooked, ½ cup	0 – 15

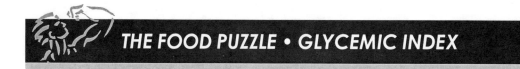
Notes on Glycemic Index

CANDIDA

Overview

Candida albicans is a type of parasitic yeast-like fungus that can inhabit the intestines, genital tract, mouth, esophagus and throat. Normally this fungus lives in balance with the other bacteria and yeasts in the body. In a healthy person a large portion of the good bacteria includes lactobacilli, which are friendly bacteria that help fight unfriendly bacteria, high cholesterol levels and even some cancers.

Unlike these good bacteria, the Candida albicans are usually only present in small numbers. They are single cell fungi that belong to the vegetable kingdom. They are cousins of the molds that live in damp basements, wood stumps and old buildings. The chart on the following page shows a visual difference between a health gut and one having an excess of yeast, parasites and/or toxins.

In a healthy body, Candida albicans are harmless. However, when certain conditions exist (such as excessive stress or lowered immune function), then this delicate balance is broken and the out-of-control fungus travels through the bloodstream to many parts of the body. It is estimated that Candida affects one out of every three Americans. This includes men and children as well as women.

Many people often mistakenly assume that if have do not have a yeast infection that they do not have Candida. This is not true, especially in the case of men. The best way to check for Candida is with the Candida questionnaire.

The most common factors contributing to Candida include:
- food allergies
- antibiotic usage
- birth control pill usage
- cortisone drugs
- infertility
- chronic fatigue
- high level consumption of caffeine and carbonated beverages
- mercury exposure via amalgam fillings and/or vaccines
- mother had Candida during pregnancy

For more detailed information on Candida, please refer to the book *Candida Made Simple* by Cheryl Townsley.

Symptom List

To determine if Candida is a problem for you, please check the following symptom list and complete the Candida questionnaire. Another method of testing for the presence of Candida is through the LFH urine test panel. One of the tests is for dysbiosis of the bowel. A positive on any of these tests is a very strong indication that Candida is present.

The following is a list of Candida symptoms. If you note that you have many of these symptoms, then Candida is highly probable.

General

- chronic fatigue
- lack of energy
- sense of poor well-being

Gastrointestinal

- dry mouth
- rash or blisters in mouth
- bad breath
- thrush (coated tongue)
- bloating, belching, intestinal gas
- intestinal cramps
- heartburn, reflux
- indigestion
- rectal itching
- diarrhea or constipation
- mucus in stools
- hemorrhoids
- irritable bowel syndrome (IBS)
- bread and/or sugar cravings

Genito-urinary

- vaginal yeast infections
- frequent bladder infections

Endocrine

- premenstrual syndrome (PMS)
- menstrual cramps
- endometriosis
- joint pain and/or swelling
- prostatitis
- loss of sex drive

Lymphatic

- post nasal drip
- sinus problems
- nasal itching
- sore and/or dry throat
- cough
- wheezing or shortness of breath
- ear pain, ringing and/or deafness
- fluid in the ears
- ear infections

Nervous System

- depression
- irritable
- brain fog
- mood swings
- frequent pains

Organs

- toxic liver
- skin problems (i.e., psoriasis, eczema hives, blemishes)
- itching
- erratic vision
- spots or floaters in eyes

Immune System

- allergies
- chemical sensitivities
- low immune function

Children's Symptoms

- ear infections
- allergies
- thrush
- mom had Candida during pregnancy

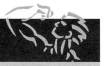

CANDIDA HISTORY & CHECKLIST FORMS

Candida Self Analysis

The following History and Major Symptom Checklist has been prepared by Lindsey Duncan, CN. and CEO of Nature's Secret. These support materials are provided based on his permission.

History – Section 1

This section involves an understanding of your medical history and how it may have promoted Candida growth. Circle the comments to which you can answer yes. Record your total at the end of the section.

Points

1. Throughout your lifetime, have you taken any antibiotics or tetracyclines (Symycin™, Panmycin™, Bivramycin™, Monicin™ etc.) for acne or other conditions, for more than one month?   25

2. Have you ever taken a "broad spectrum" antibiotic for more than two months or four or more times in a one-year period? These could include any antibiotics taken for respiratory, urinary or other infections.   20

3. Have you taken a "broad spectrum" antibiotic – even for a single course? These antibiotics include ampicillin™, amoxicillin™, Keflex™, etc.   (6)

4. Have you ever had problems with persistent prostatitis, vaginitis or other problems with your reproductive organs?   25

5. Women – Have you been pregnant:
   Two or more times?   (5)
   One time?   3

6. Women – Have you taken birth control pills:
   More than two years?   15
   More than six months?   (8)

7. If you were not breast-fed as an infant.   9

8. Have you taken any cortisone-type drugs (Prednisone™, Decadron™, etc.)?   15

9. Are you sensitive to and bothered by exposure to perfumes, insecticides or other chemical odors:
   Do you have moderate to severe symptoms?   20
   Do you have mild symptoms?   5

Points

10. Does tobacco smoke bother you? (10)

11. Are your symptoms worse on damp, muggy days or in moldy places? 20

12. If you have had chronic fungus infections of the skin or nails
    (including athlete's foot, ring worm, jock itch), have the infections been:
    Severe or persistent? 20
    Mild to moderate? 10

13. Do you crave sugar (chocolate, ice cream, candy, cookies, etc.)? 10

14. Do you crave carbohydrates (bread, bread and more bread)? (10)

15. Do you crave alcoholic beverages? 10

16. Have you drunk or do you drink chlorinated water (city or tap)? (20)

Total Score Section 1 ___59___

Major Symptoms – Section 2

For each of your symptoms, enter the appropriate figure in the point score column.

No symptoms	0
Occasional or mild	3
Frequent and/or moderately severe	6
Severe and/or disabling	9

Points

1. Constipation ___0___

2. Diarrhea ___0___

3. Bloating ___3___

4. Fatigue or lethargy ___0___

5. Feeling drained ___0___

		Points
6.	Poor memory	3
7.	Difficulty focusing/brain fog	3
8.	Feeling moody or despair	3
9.	Numbness, burning or tingling	0
10.	Muscle aches	0
11.	Nasal congestion or discharge	0
12.	Pain and/or swelling in the joints	0
13.	Abdominal pain	0
14.	Spots in front of the eyes	0
15.	Erratic vision	0
16.	Cold hands and/or feet	6

Women

17.	Endometriosis	0
18.	Menstrual irregularities and/or severe cramps	0
19.	PMS	3
20.	Vaginal discharge	0
21.	Persistent vaginal burning or itching	0

Men

22.	Prostatitis	——
23.	Impotence	——

Women and Men

24.	Loss of sexual desire	6

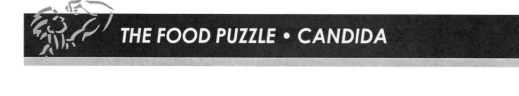
	Points
25. Low blood sugar	0
26. Anger or frustration	0
27. Dry, patchy skin	0

Total Score Section 2 __27__

Minor Symptoms – Section 3

For each of your symptoms, enter the appropriate figure in the point score column.

No symptoms	0
Occasional or mild	1
Frequent and/or moderately severe	2
Severe and/or disabling	3

	Points
1. Heartburn	0
2. Indigestion	0
3. Belching and intestinal gas	0
4. Drowsiness	0
5. Itching	0
6. Rashes	0
7. Irritability or jitters	0
8. Uncoordinated	0
9. Inability to concentrate	1
10. Frequent mood swings	0

Points

11. Postnasal drip	0
12. Nasal itching	0
13. Failing vision	0
14. Burning or tearing of the eyes	0
15. Recurrent infections of fluid in the ears	0
16. Ear pain or deafness	0
17. Headaches	0
18. Dizziness/loss of balance	0
19. Pressure above the ears (your head feels like it is swelling and tingling)	0
20. Mucus in the stool	0
21. Hemorrhoids	0
22. Dry mouth	0
23. Rash or blisters in the mouth	1
24. Bad breath	1
25. Sore or dry throat	0
26. Cough	0
27. Pain or tightness in the chest	0
28. Wheezing or shortness of breath	0
29. Urinary urgency or frequency	1
30. Burning during urination	0

Total Score Section 3 ____4____

The Results

Total Score from Section 1   59

Total Score from Section 2   27

Total Score from Section 3   4

Total Score   90

If your score is at least:	*Your symptoms are:*
180 Women	Almost certainly yeast connected
140 Men	Almost certainly yeast connected

▲ ▼ ▲ ▼ ▲ ▼ ▲ ▼ ▲ ▼ ▲ ▼ ▲ ▼ ▲

120 Women	Probably yeast connected
90 Men	Probably yeast connected

90   ▲ ▼ ▲ ▼ ▲ ▼ ▲ ▼ ▲ ▼ ▲ ▼ ▲ ▼ ▲

60 Women	Possibly yeast connected
40 Men	Possibly yeast connected

▲ ▼ ▲ ▼ ▲ ▼ ▲ ▼ ▲ ▼ ▲ ▼ ▲ ▼ ▲

If your score is less than:	*Your symptoms are:*
60 Women	Probably not yeast connected
40 Men	Probably not yeast connected

If your score is 60+ (women) or 40+ (men), then you will probably want to consider following the suggestions found in this book.

How to do a Candida Cleanse

The following protocol covers the basic steps of a Candida cleanse. A Candida cleanse is not harmful if done without the presence of Candida. This type of cleanse is good for parasites and overall health of the bowel. A Candida cleanse, done at least once per year, is good insurance in building a healthy colon – I do one at least once each year. For more support or a customized program, you can work with a LFH Coach or your health care practitioner.

Cleanse Protocol

When doing a cleanse, five steps must be followed. The *first step* to a successful cleanse is the diet. The standard American diet (SAD) is the culprit for much of the Candida problem. To eliminate Candida those foods that feed Candida must be removed in order to stop the food chain that is feeding the Candida. A Candida cleanse should be done for at least one month and up to six months, depending on the severity and length of your condition.

The *second step* includes herbal and/or homeopathic support to kill the Candida. Just as important as removing the food that feeds the fungus is the herbal support necessary to destroy the fungus and help restore normal bowel environment.

In our clinical practice we have noted that all blood types do well on a herbal cleanse. However, where there is a highly toxic liver due to chemical exposures and/or high levels of mercury/amalgam fillings, a homeopathic remedy that also supports liver drainage can be more successful. If in doubt, start with the herbal program. If you do not experience noticeable differences in one month, then see your health care provider or a LFH Coach.

The *third step* is the removal of those offenders that help set the stage for fungal overgrowth. Those items include overuse/misuse of oral antibiotics, food containing antibiotics (much of our commercial meat, dairy and farm raised fish), birth control pills and steroids. If you are taking any of these items under the direction of your physician, please check with him/her before stopping.

The *fourth step* is the bowel support process. It is essential to supply the body with good enzymes, probiotics and essential fatty acids, in order to restore a healthy bowel terrain. Without these supports both during and after a cleanse, it is highly unlikely that you will achieve long term success. You must create a bowel environment that is "unfriendly" to Candida and "friendly" to the healthy bacteria.

The *fifth step* is ongoing lifestyle changes. Your current diet and lifestyle choices have created your current health challenges. In order to avoid a reoccurrence, permanent changes need to be made. Those changes include following your Food Puzzle, avoiding refined foods, taking the cell essential nutrients in a daily smoothie and the regular use of enzymes and probiotics. Fiber is necessary if you tend towards constipation. The purpose of *Body by Design* is to help you make those changes, step by step, in such a way that *they become a permanent and normal part of your life.*

Step One: Omit the Food that Feeds Candida

Certain foods feed fungus. Consuming these foods during a cleanse slows the healing process and feeds the offenders – the fungus. The more of these foods you eliminate, the more successful your cleanse will be in a shorter period of time. The least amount of time to eliminate these foods is one month. It may be necessary to continue this diet for a longer period of time if the fungus overgrowth is severe.

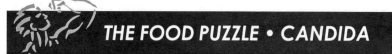

Even if you cannot totally eliminate the following foods, you will experience benefit for each food you do eliminate, especially white sugar, white flour and white rice. These highly refined foods impact Candida as well as the overall function of the immune system.

Be sure to read labels closely. You will be surprised how many of these foods are in packaged foods. For example, vinegar is in ketchup, mustard, mayonnaise, pickles and many salad dressings. Don't assume – read the labels!

Foods to Avoid:
- refined sugar, fruit, fruit juice, honey, fructose, maple syrup, other sweeteners
- yeast (i.e., bread and all foods containing yeast)
- alcohol (especially beer and wine) and caffeine (coffee and chocolate)
- dairy products, especially cheese
- fermented foods (i.e., vinegar, tofu, soy sauce, tamari)
- wheat (whole wheat and white flour)
- dried fruits
- peanuts
- white rice
- allergenic foods (see your food puzzle "omit" foods)
- mushrooms

As you read this list you may feel you have nothing left to eat! The problem with most people who have Candida is that the above list is what they eat, what they crave and what feeds their problem. The cravings are an indication of the presence of the fungus and the established routine of feeding the fungus.

Following a Candida cleanse, you will be able to add fruit, cider vinegar (if tolerated – as indicated by your Food Puzzle), tamari, whole wheat (if tolerated), dried fruits and whole grain breads back into your diet. Long term success will require staying off of the whites – flour, sugar, rice – as well as most dairy products.

There are many foods left to eat. Check out the beneficial and neutral foods later in this book and learn to enjoy them. For ideas on how to prepare many of these foods, I recommend the *Lifestyle for Health Cookbook* and the *Candida Control Cookbook* (see order form).

For a natural sweetener for beverages, I recommend using stevia. Stevia is an herb that has no effect on blood sugar and is safe for diabetics. The liquid form works well for cooking, beverages and other uses. One teaspoon of the liquid is equivalent to one cup of refined sugar. For cooking with stevia, I recommend *Stevia Sweet Recipes,* a stevia cookbook (see order form).

Step 2: Use a Candida Cleanse Product
For the average person, a cleanse that contains anti-fungal herbs is best. The herbs that are best for Candida include:
- garlic
- pau d'arco
- barberry root
- olive leaf

- clove bud
- peppermint leaf
- uva ursi

Be sure to follow the directions on the package of a Candida cleanse for maximum results. For product recommendations of Candida cleanses please see page 96.

If you have significant mercury fillings and/or chemical exposures, it is recommended that you support the liver. If you do an herbal cleanse and have any problem or do not get results, this is when you need to work with a professional. Yeast can be persistent in a body that is loaded with heavy metal toxicity and chemical toxicity. A qualified practitioner can help you with this situation or you can work with a LFH Coach.

I have found that homeopathic cleanses work best for children and for people who have trouble swallowing pills. A homeopathic cleanse is also helpful when a person has had high exposure to chemicals and/or currently has significant amounts of silver/amalgam fillings. A homeopathic cleanse that includes liver drainage for these chemical toxins is more helpful for blood type Os and Bs than the other blood types.

If a child can swallow pills and is over the age of ten, then I recommend the parents use a cleanse that is especially formulated for children, such as ParaGone for Kids by Advanced Naturals. This cleanse addresses both parasites (often an issue if you have pets, travel and/or eat out) and fungus.

Step 3: Reduce Stressors

The most significant stressors on the body that add to the Candida problem should also be eliminated where possible. Antibiotics, birth control pills and steroids feed fungal problems. *Be sure to check with your doctor before eliminating any of these items.*

Stressful lifestyles compromise the immune system. Most people are aware of stress but are unsure of how to address it. Eating a healthier diet is a first good step. Two other easily used strategies are the "4-2-4" and the "trip to Tahiti."

The "4-2-4" is the rhythm for deep breathing. Breathing in through the nose, breathe in deeply to the count of four. Hold for the count of two and then slowly breathe out through the nose to the count of four. Doing this several times during the day is a great de-stressor.

The "trip to Tahiti" exercise was presented during a class I attended by Apex. In this exercise you need to lay flat on the floor with arms at the side of the body. Place the feet and lower legs up on the seat of a chair. The legs will be bent at the knee and the body will be on the floor. With no music, no distraction, close your eyes and rest. Fifteen minutes in this position can offer as much rest and relaxation as an eight-hour sleep. For people under high stress, this should be done twice a day.

In addition to these exercises, it is recommended that you include an adrenal supplement to help you handle the stress on the adrenals. For recommended adrenal supplementation check with your health care provider or you can check the recommendations at the end of the book. Testing by your health care provider or through the LFH Urine Test Panel is highly recommended to ensure the most appropriate support is being used.

A simple way to reduce dietary stress (in addition to following your *Food Puzzle*!) is to slow down and chew slowly. Gulping your food inhibits digestive juices in the mouth to break down food for the rest of the digestive system. The American way of "gulping and inhaling" food is one of the worst stressors on the body. Slow down, enjoy your food and take time for conversation. Your tummy will love you for the change!

Consuming large amounts of water during a meal also inhibits proper digestion. It is best to consume your water before a meal or about an hour or two after a meal. If you do consume beverages during a meal, please sip and consume as small an amount as possible.

Being thirsty during a meal is often a sign of dehydration. Consuming more water during the day will help. Many beverages consumed are actually diuretics. Coffee, black tea and other caffeinated beverages are the worst for dehydrating the body. Avoid coffee, black tea and soda as much as possible to improve digestion and overall health.

Step 4: Include Digestive Support

Since poorly digested food adds to the problem, digestive support can be helpful. The easiest way to determine the best enzyme support for your digestive system is to take the Enzyme Questionnaire (found later in this book). Total the scores by section. You can take up to three enzymes for which you have the highest scores. Be sure to take these enzymes according to the directions on the bottle – recommendations include before, between and/or after meals. No more than three enzymes solutions should be taken without the direction of your health care provider or a LFH Coach.

A natural way to get enzymes is through juicing. Juicing removes the fiber, but concentrates the natural enzymes found in fresh fruits and vegetables. While on a Candida cleanse, the juicing should primarily be green vegetables and a very small amount of Granny Smith apples or carrots for flavor (preferably organic). Green veggies are rich in nitrogen, enzymes and many other healing properties. Be careful not to juice only carrots and/or fruit during a Candida cleanse as they can feed the problem, due to their high sugar content.

Probiotics are essential during and after a Candida cleanse. Probiotics are friendly, beneficial bacteria that help fight fungus (as well as bacteria and parasite overgrowth) and restore proper bacteria balance to the intestinal tract. The two most important categories of good bacteria are lactobacillus acidophilus and bifidobacterium bifidum. Probiotics should be taken on an empty stomach for maximum benefit.

The reason probiotics need to be used following a cleanse is that many uncontrollable aspects of our environment and lifestyle are continually at work to upset this bacteria balance. Stress, processed foods, medications, caffeine, cigarette smoke and chemical exposures are not always controllable. By controlling the stressors that you can and by taking probiotics for those that you can't, you are helping to ensure optimal health in the colon.

Step 5: Maintenance

Once you have completed a Candida cleanse and no longer have an overgrowth of yeast (this can be confirmed by your health care practitioner or by taking the LFH urine test panel), it is important to follow good maintenance procedures to keep the problem from returning.

The best way to determine your progress is to note changes in the symptoms you observed at the beginning of the cleanse. For example, if you experienced fatigue before the cleanse and are now experiencing increased energy then you are improving. If you stop the cleanse at this point and fatigue reappears then you have stopped the cleanse prematurely. It is recommended that you resume the cleanse for another month.

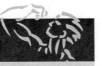

The following elements are key for any maintenance plan following a Candida cleanse:

- avoid the stressors and diet that caused the problem in the first place
- support your immune system on a daily basis with the essential cell builders found in the LFH smoothie recipe
- take a good quality garlic
- daily use of probiotics
- include appropriate enzyme support (according to your enzyme questionnaire)
- include fiber – either dietary or supplemental (be sure to follow directions and consume plenty of water)
- daily exercise (recommend rebounding)

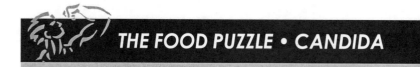

Notes on Candida

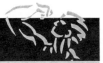

BLOOD TYPE

What Is Blood Type?

Our blood contains chemical markers called antigens, which are in every cell of our bodies. One of the most powerful antigens in humans is the one that determines your blood type. These various antigens are so powerful, that when operating efficiently, they represent a key part of the immune system. When your immune system senses a foreign element (i.e., bacteria, virus, fungus, etc.), it looks to the blood type antigen to know if the element is friend or foe.

Each blood type possesses its unique antigen with its own chemical structure. These structures are antennae lying on the cell membranes of the blood cells. These antennae are comprised of long chains of sugars and each blood type has a different blend of these glyconutrients.

- Blood Type O   contains fucose
- Blood Type A   contains fucose (O's sugar) and N-acetyl-galactosamine
- Blood Type B   contains fucose (O's sugar) and D-galactosamine
- Blood Type AB contains fucose (O's sugar), N-acetyl-galactosamine (A's sugar) and
                                          D-galactosamine (B's sugar)

As a result of these sugars, each person has a specific set of antigens working to build the immune system. Because of these different antigens, each of us is susceptible to different food challenges when we eat. Every food is made of different lectins (proteins). These lectins interact differently with each blood type. When there is a negative interaction, it interferes with your digestion, metabolism and immune system. How this interaction occurs is covered, in great detail, by Dr. Peter J. D'Adamo in his books *Eat Right for Your Blood Type* and *Live Right for Your Type*.

By avoiding the negative foods for your blood type you reduce stress on your digestive and immune systems, freeing up vital energy that can now manifest as health, vitality and energy!

Please note that our *Food Puzzle* recommendations are guidelines, not rules. As you work with your specific guidelines, please remember that you may need to make some adjustments to best fit your unique makeup.

Determining Blood Type

To determine your blood type, ask your doctor to check your medical records. Blood typing from your doctor is not covered by insurance and is usually billed in excess of $200.00. You can also determine your blood type when you donate blood. LFH has blood type kits for self testing at home. (See the order form at the back of this book.) This simple at home test takes less than three minutes and comes with complete directions. You will need one kit per person.

Unclean Foods

The following foods are biblically unclean foods and therefore not included in any of the food lists.

Unclean Meats

Ostrich	Rabbit
Pork	Squirrel

Unclean Fish

Blowfish	Lobster	Shark
Catfish	Octopus	Shrimp
Crab	Puffer	Sturgeon
Eel	Sea squab	Swordfish

Blood Type O

The foods that have a "†" notation indicate foods that cause a high glycemic response. These foods should be omitted in order to lose fat.

If you have Candida, omit the foods that are *italicized* during a Candida cleanse. After the cleanse, or if you do not have Candida, use the foods accordingly.

Beneficial Foods • Blood Type O

Proteins • Beneficial • Blood Type O
Meat

If you are a Profile 1 or Slow Burner, please read the Metabolic Profile section before applying this information.

Beef	Lamb	Venison
Beef: ground	Organ meats	
Buffalo	Veal	

Seafood

Bluefish	Rainbow trout	Yellowtail
Cod	Salmon	
Hake	Sardine	
Halibut	Snapper: all, red	
Mackerel	Sole	
Perch: white, yellow	Striped bass	
Pike	Whitefish	

Dairy and Eggs

None

Beans and Peas

Aduke	Black-eyed peas
Azuki	Pinto

Fats • Beneficial • Blood Type O
Oils

Flaxseed oil	Olive oil

Nuts and Seeds

Pumpkin seeds	Walnuts

Carbohydrates • Beneficial • Blood Type O
Cereals

None

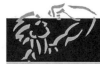

Breads and Muffins

Sprouted grain products, such as:

Alverado	*Ezekial*
Essene	*Manna*

Grains and Pasta

None

Vegetables • Beneficial • Blood Type O

Artichokes	Horseradish	Parsnips†
Beet leaves	Kale	Peppers: red
Broccoli	Kohlrabi	Potatoes: sweet
Chicory	Leek	Pumpkin†
Collard greens	Lettuce: romaine	Seaweed
Dandelion	Okra	Spinach
Escarole	Onions: red, Spanish, yellow	Swiss chard
Garlic	Parsley	Turnips†

Fruits • Beneficial • Blood Type O

Figs	*Plums*	*Prunes*

Juices • Beneficial • Blood Type O

Black cherry	*Pineapple*	*Prune*

Spices • Beneficial • Blood Type O

Carob	Dulse	Turmeric
Cayenne	Kelp	
Curry	Parsley	

Condiments • Beneficial • Blood Type O

None

Herbs and Teas • Beneficial • Blood Type O

Cayenne	Hops	Rose hips
Chickweed	Linden	Sarsaparilla
Dandelion	Mulberry	Slippery elm
Fenugreek	Parsley	
Ginger	Peppermint	

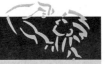

Neutral Foods • Blood Type O

Protein • Neutral • Blood Type O

Meat

Chicken	Partridge	Quail
Cornish Hen	Pheasant	
Duck	Turkey	

Seafood

Albacore (tuna)	Flounder	Perch: Ocean
Anchovy	Haddock	
Bluegill bass	Mahi-mahi	

Dairy and Eggs

Butter	*Feta*	Soy cheese and milk need
Eggs	*Goat cheese*	to be tested.
Farmer cheese	*Mozzarella*	

Beans and Peas

Black	Green beans	Red
Broad†	Green peas, pea pods	Snap
Cannellini	Jicama	String
Fava†	Lima	White
Garbanzo	Northern	

Fats • Neutral • Blood Type O

Oils

Canola	Cod liver	Sesame

Nuts and Seeds

Almonds	Hickory	Sesame: butter, seeds
Almond butter	Macadamia	Sunflower: seeds, butter
Chestnuts	Pecans	
Filberts	Pine nuts	

Carbohydrates • Neutral • Blood Type O

Cereals

Amaranth	Cream of rice†	Millet†
Barley	*Kamut*	Rice: bran, puffed†
Buckwheat	Kasha†	*Spelt*

Breads

Brown rice	Rice cakes†	Wheat-free bread

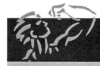

Breads, continued

Fin crisp†	Rye bread: 100%†	Wasa bread
Kamut bread	*Spelt bread*	

Grains and Pasta

Artichoke pasta	Kasha†	Rye flour†
Barley flour	Quinoa	*Spelt flour*
Buckwheat	Rice: basmati, brown, wild	

Vegetables • Neutral • Blood Type O

Aarugula	Lettuce	Scallions
Asparagus	Lima beans	Shallots
Bamboo shoots	Mushrooms: enoki,	Snow peas
Beets	portobello, oyster	Sprouts: mung, radish
Bok choy	Olives: green	Squash: all
Caraway	Onions: green	Tomato
Carrots†	Peppers: green,	Water chestnuts
Celery	yellow, jalapeno	Yams: all
Cucumber	Radicchio	Zucchini
Daikon	Radishes	Test all soy products.
Endive	Rappini	
Ginger	Rutabaga†	

Fruits • Neutral • Blood Type O

Apples	*Grapes*	*Papayas*
Apricots	*Guava*	*Peaches*
Bananas	*Kiwi*	*Pears*
Blueberries	*Kumquat*	*Persimmons*
Boysenberries	*Lemons*	*Pineapples*
Cherries	*Limes*	*Pomegranates*
Cranberries	*Loganberries*	*Prickly pear*
Currants	*Mangoes*	*Raisins*
Dates†	*Melon: casaba, crenshaw,*	*Raspberries*
Elderberries	*Christmas, musk,*	*Starfruit*
Gooseberries	*watermelon†*	
Grapefruit	*Nectarines*	

Juices • Neutral • Blood Type O

Apricot	*Cranberry*	*Grapefruit*
Carrot†	*Cucumber*	Vegetables (As
Celery	*Grape*	shown in above category.)

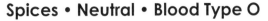

Spices • Neutral • Blood Type O

Agar	Cumin	Pimento
Allspice	Dill	Pimiento
Almond extract	Garlic	Rice syrup
Anise	Gelatin: plain	Rosemary
Arrowroot	*Honey†*	Saffron
Barley malt	Horseradish	Sage
Basil	*Maple syrup†*	Salt: sea, Real™
Bay leaf	Marjoram	Savory
Brown rice syrup	Mint	Spearmint
Cardamom	*Miso*	*Sucanat†*
Chervil	*Molasses†*	*Tamari*
Chives	Mustard: dry	Tamarind
Chocolate	Paprika	Tapioca
Clove	Pepper: peppercorn,	Tarragon
Coriander	red flakes	Thyme
Cream of tartar	Peppermint	Wintergreen

Condiments • Neutral • Blood Type O

Apple butter	*Mayonnaise*	*Worcestershire*
Jam	*Mustard*	

Herbs and Teas • Neutral • Blood Type O

Catnip	Horehound	Thyme
Chamomile	Licorice root	Valerian
Dong quai	Mullein	Vervain
Elder	Raspberry leaf	White birch
Ginseng	Sage	White oak bark
Green tea	Skullcap	Yarrow
Hawthorn	Spearmint	

Foods to Avoid • Blood Type O

Protein • Avoid • Blood Type O

Meat

Unclean meats – pork, goose

Seafood

Barracuda	Conch	Octopus
Catfish	Herring	Unclean fish
Caviar	Lox	

Dairy and Eggs

American	Edam	Provolone
Blue cheese	Emmenthal	Neufchatel
Brie	Gouda	Ricotta
Buttermilk	Gruyere	Skim milk: 2%
Camembert	Ice cream	String cheese
Casein	Jarlsberg	Swiss
Cheddar	Kefir	Whey
Colby cheese	Monterey	Whole milk
Cottage	Munster	Yogurt: all
Cream cheese	Parmesan	

Beans and Legumes

Copper	Navy
Kidney	Lentils: domestic, green, red

Fats • Avoid • Blood Type O

Oils

Corn	Peanut
Cottonseed	Safflower

Nuts and Seeds

Brazil	Litchi	Pistachio
Cashews	Peanuts, peanut butter	Poppy seeds

Carbohydrates • Avoid • Blood Type O

Cereals

Cornflakes	Farina	Seven-grain
Cornmeal	Grape nuts	Shredded wheat
Cream of wheat	Oat bran	Wheat: bran, germ
Familia	Oatmeal	

Breads

Bagels	Matzos	Wheat bran bread
Corn muffins	Multi-grain bread	Wheat bran muffins
English muffins	Oat bran muffins	Wheat: durum, whole
High-protein bread	Pumpernickel	

Grains and Pasta

Bulgur wheat	Graham flour	Soba noodles
Couscous	Oat flour	Wheat flour
Durum wheat	Pasta: semolina, spinach	White flour

Vegetables • Avoid • Blood Type O

Avocado
Brussels sprouts
Cabbage: Chinese, red, white
Cauliflower

Corn: white, yellow
Eggplant
Mushrooms: domestic, shitake

Mustard greens
Olives: black, Greek, Spanish
Potatoes: red, white
Sprouts: alfalfa

Fruits • Avoid • Blood Type O

Blackberries
Coconut
Melon: cantaloupe, honeydew

Oranges
Plantains
Rhubarb

Strawberries
Tangerines

Juices • Avoid • Blood Type O

Apple

Cabbage

Orange

Spices • Avoid • Blood Type O

Capers
Cinnamon
Cornstarch

Corn syrup
Nutmeg
Pepper: black ground

Vanilla
Vinegar: apple cider, balsamic, red, white

Condiments • Avoid • Blood Type O

Ketchup

Pickles

Pickle relish

Herbs and Teas • Avoid • Blood Type O

Alfalfa
Aloe
Burdock
Coltsfoot
Corn silk

Echinacea
Gentian
Goldenseal
Red clover
Rhubarb

St. John's Wort
Senna
Shepherd's Purse
Yellow Dock

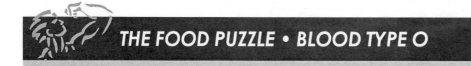

Blood Type O Summary Information

Strengths

- stronger digestive systems
- stronger immune systems
- risk taker
- leader

Common Emotional issues

- anger/shame
- grief/sadness
- type A personalities, perfectionism
- insensitive to others

Physical Weaknesses

- weaker to dental and chemical toxicity
- tends to have stressed lungs, liver and/or adrenals

Exercise

- intense exertion
- rebounding
- resistance training
- aerobics
- martial arts
- contact sports
- running

Weight Loss Tips

- omit wheat and corn from the diet as they impact insulin efficiency and slow metabolic function
- avoid kidney beans and lentils as they impair calorie utilization
- avoid cabbage, Brussels sprouts, cauliflower and mustard greens as they can inhibit thyroid function
- can handle higher levels of metabolic acidity
- monitor thyroid function (usually need to avoid soy)
- ensure adequate levels of iodine (practitioner can assess iodine levels)

Common Diseases and Suggestions

ADD, ADHD

- exercise
- essential fatty acids (EFAs)
- avoid wheat and dairy

Allergies (i.e., chemical, wheat, corn, dairy) – may manifest as Candida
- omit allergenic foods
- if Candida shows – support the liver and eliminate the fungus with homeopathics or herbs
- heavy metal and liver cleanses

Asthma, Hayfever
- check for allergies and/or food sensitivities
- lung and/or adrenal support
- lymph drainers, especially a mucus drainer

Blood Clotting Disorder
- blood purifiers
- lymph drainers

CFS
- check for toxic liver
- support adrenals

Chron's or Celiac Sprue
- avoid wheat
- probiotics
- enzymes

Diarrhea
- often a reaction to dairy and/or wheat
- probiotics
- enzymes

Inflammatory Diseases such as Arthritis
- glucosamine, chondrotin
- avoid nightshades (potatoes, peppers, eggplant)
- vitamin C (avoid ascorbic acid if pH is acid)

Low Thyroid Production
- iodine sources (kelp)
- seafood

Ulcers
- enzymes
- check for hydrochloric acid levels (see vinegar test at end), add HCL if levels are low
- de-glycyrrhizinated licorice (DGL licorice) can help with excess stomach acid

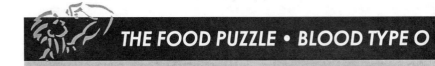
Best Nutrients for Blood Type O

- cell essentials – smoothie
- vitamin B (a B complex, not B-12 or folic acid, unless identified by health care practitioner)
- pancreatic enzymes, protease or enzymes for added protein metabolism
- calcium (monitor this based on pH levels), non-dairy sources
- iodine or kelp for thyroid support, as needed
- manganese
- avoid added vitamin A and E as they tend to thin blood too much for an O
- heavy metal and liver cleanses

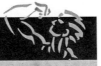

Blood Type A

The foods that have a "†" notation indicate foods that cause a high glycemic response. These foods should be omitted in order to lose fat.

If you have Candida, omit the foods that are *italicized* during a Candida cleanse. After the cleanse, or if you do not have Candida, use the foods accordingly.

Beneficial Foods • Blood Type A

Proteins • Beneficial • Blood Type A

Meat

If you are a Profile 2 or Fast Burner, please read the Metabolic Profile section before applying this information.
None

Seafood

Cod	Pickerel	Sea trout
Grouper	Rainbow trout	Snapper: red
Mackerel	Salmon	Whitefish
Perch: silver, yellow	Sardine	

Dairy and Eggs

Soy: cheese, milk

Beans and Legumes

Aduke	Green	Peas: black-eyes
Azuki	Pinto	Red soy
Black	Lentils: domestic, green, red	

Fats • Beneficial • Blood Type A

Oils

Flaxseed	Olive

Nuts and Seeds

Peanuts, peanut butter‡   Pumpkin seeds
‡Can be high in mold.

Carbohydrates • Beneficial • Blood Type A

Cereals

Amaranth	Buckwheat	Kasha†

Breads

Sprouted: Alvarado,   Rice cakes†
Essene, Ezekial, Manna

Grains and Pasta

Artichoke pasta

Buckwheat kasha

Flour: oat†, rice†, rye†

Soba noodles

Vegetables • Beneficial • Blood Type A

Artichokes

Beet leaves

Broccoli

Carrots†

Chicory

Collard greens

Dandelion

Escarole

Garlic

Horseradish

Kale

Kohlrabi

Leek

Lettuce: romaine

Okra

Onions: red, Spanish, yellow

Parsley

Parsnips†

Pumpkin†

Spinach

Sprouts: alfalfa

Swiss Chard

Tempeh

Tofu

Turnips†

Fruits • Beneficial • Blood Type A

Apricots

Blackberries

Blueberries

Boysenberries

Cherries

Cranberries

Figs

Grapefruit

Lemons

Pineapple

Plums

Prunes

Raisins

Juices • Beneficial • Blood Type A

Apricot

Carrot†

Celery

Cherry: black

Grapefruit

Pineapple

Prune

Water with lemon

Spices • Beneficial • Blood Type A

Barley malt†

Blackstrap molasses†

Garlic

Ginger

Miso

Tamari

Condiments • Beneficial • Blood Type A

Mustard

Herbs and Teas • Beneficial • Blood Type A

Alfalfa

Aloe

Burdock

Chamomile

Echinacea

Fenugreek

Ginger

Ginseng

Green tea

Hawthorn

Milk Thistle

Rose Hips

St. John's Wort

Slippery Elm

Valerian

Neutral Foods • Blood Type A

Protein • Neutral • Blood Type A

Meats

If you are a Profile 2 or Fast Burner, please read the Metabolic Profile section before applying this information.

Chicken	Cornish hens	Turkey

Seafood

Albacore (tuna)	Pike	Yellowtail
Mahi-mahi	Sea bass	
Perch: ocean, white	Snapper	

Dairy and Eggs

Eggs	*Goat: cheese, milk*	*Ricotta*
Farmer cheese	*Kefir*	*String cheese*
Feta	*Mozzarella*	*Yogurt: all*

Beans and Legumes

Broad†	Jicama	String
Cannelini	Peas: green, pods, snow	White
Fava†	Snap	

Fats • Neutral • Blood Type A

Oils

Canola	Cod liver

Nuts and Seeds

Almonds, almond butter	Litchi	Sesame: butter, seeds
Chestnuts	Macadamia	Sunflower: seeds, butter
Filberts	Pine nuts	Walnuts
Hickory	Poppy seeds	

Carbohydrates • Neutral • Blood Type A

Cereals

Barley	Cream of rice†	Oat: bran, oatmeal
Cornflakes†	*Kamut*	Rice: bran, whole†, brown†
Cornmeal†	Millet†	*Spelt*

Breads

Bagels: whole wheat†	Gluten-free bread†	*Spelt*
Brown rice bread†	*Kamut bread*	Wasa bread
Corn muffins†	Millet†	

Breads, continued

Fin crisp†   *Rye: 100%†*

Grains and Pasta

Couscous†   Pasta: brown rice†, spelt, kamut

Flour: barley, bulgur, *wheat†,*   Quinoa

   durum†, gluten†, graham†   Rice: basmati, brown, wild

   spelt, sprouted wheat

Vegetables • Neutral • Blood Type A

Aragula	Cucumber	Radicchio
Asparagus	Daikon radish	Radishes
Avocado	Endive	Rappini
Bamboo shoots	Fennel	Rutabaga†
Beets	Ginger	Scallions
Bok choy	Lettuce: all	Seaweed
Brussels Sprouts	*Mushroom: enoki,*	Shallots
Caraway	*portobello, oyster*	Sprouts: all
Cauliflower	Mustard greens	Squash: all
Celery	Olive: green	Water chestnut
Chervil	Onions: green	Watercress
Corn†	Pumpkin†	Zucchini

Fruits • Neutral • Blood Type A

Apples	*Kumquat*	*Peaches*
Currants	*Limes*	*Pears*
Dates†	*Loganberries*	*Persimmons*
Elderberries	*Melon: casaba, crenshaw,*	*Pomegranates*
Gooseberries	*musk, Spanish,*	*Prickly pear*
Grapes: all	*watermelon†*	*Starfruit*
Guava	*Nectarines*	*Strawberries*
Kiwi		

Juices • Neutral • Blood Type A

Apple	*Cucumber*	*Grape*
Cabbage	*Cranberry*	Vegetable (from Neutral list)

Spices • Neutral • Blood Type A

Agar	Corn: starch, syrup†	Peppermint
Allspice	Cream of tartar	Pimento
Almond extract	Cumin	*Rice syrup†*
Anise	Curry	Rosemary
Arrowroot	Dill	Saffron

Spices • Neutral • Blood Type A, continued

Basil	*Honey†*	Sage
Bay leaf	Horseradish	Salt: sea, Real™
Brown rice syrup†	Kelp	Savory
Cardamom	*Maple syrup†*	Spearmint
Carob	Marjoram	*Sucanat†*
Chervil	Mint	Tamarind
Chives	Mustard: dry	Tapioca
Chocolate	Nutmeg	Tarragon
Cinnamon	Oregano	Thyme
Cloves	Paprika	Turmeric
Coriander	Parsley	Vanilla

Condiments • Neutral • Blood Type A

Pickles: dill, kosher, sweet, sour

Herbs and Tea • Neutral • Blood Type A

Chickweed	Linden	Skullcap
Coltsfoot	Mulberry	Spearmint
Dandelion	Mullein	Strawberry leaf
Dong quai	Parsley	Thyme
Elder	Peppermint	Vervain
Gentian	Raspberry leaf	White birch
Goldenseal	Sage	White oak bark
Hops	Sarsaparilla	Yarrow
Horehound	Senna	
Licorice root	Shepherd's purse	

Foods to Avoid • Blood Type A

Proteins • Avoid • Blood Type A

Meats

If you are a Profile 2 or Fast Burner, please read the Metabolic Profile section before applying this information.

Beef	Goose	Veal
Buffalo	Organ meats	Venison
Duck	Unclean meats	

Seafood

Anchovy	Caviar	Lox
Beluga	Flounder	Unclean seafood
Bluefish	Haddock	
Bluegill bass	Halibut	

Dairy and Eggs

American cheese	Cottage cheese	Neufchatel
Blue cheese	Edam	Parmesan
Brie	Emmenthal	Provolone
Butter	Gouda	Sherbet
Buttermilk	Gruyere	Swiss
Camembert	Ice cream	Whey
Casein	Jarlsburg	
Cheddar	Milk: skim, 2%, whole	
Colby	Monterey jack	
Cream cheese	Munster	

Beans and Legumes

Copper	Lima	Tamarind
Garbanzo	Navy	
Kidney	Red	

Fats • Avoid • Blood Type A

Oils

Corn	Peanut	Sesame
Cottonseed	Safflower	

Nuts and Seeds

Brazil	Cashew	Pistachios

Carbohydrates • Avoid • Blood Type A

Cereals

Cream of wheat	Granola	Shredded wheat
Familia	Grape nuts	Wheat: bran, germ, whole
Farina	Seven-grain	

Breads

English muffins	Matzos	Pumpernickel
High-protein bread	Multi-grain bread	Wheat: muffins, bread

Grains and Pastas

Flour: wheat	Pasta: semolina, spinach

Vegetables • Avoid • Blood Type A

Cabbage: all	Mushrooms: shitake	Potatoes: sweet, red, white
Eggplant	Olives: black, Greek,	Tomatoes
Lima beans	Spanish	Yams
Mushrooms: domestic,	Peppers: all	

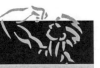

Fruits • Avoid • Blood Type A

Bananas	Oranges	Tangerines
Coconuts	Papayas	
Mangoes	Plantains	
Melon: cantaloupe, honeydew	Rhubarb	

Juices • Avoid • Blood Type A

Orange	Papaya	Tomato

Spices • Avoid • Blood Type A

Capers	Pepper: all	Wintergreen
Gelatin: plain	Vinegar: all	

Condiments • Avoid • Blood Type A

Ketchup	Mayonnaise	Worcestershire sauce

Herbs and Tea • Avoid • Blood Type A

Catnip	Corn silk	Rhubarb
Cayenne	Red clover	Yellow dock

Blood Type A Summary Information

Strengths

- adapts to environmental changes
- spiritually, emotionally and physically sensitive
- metabolizes nutrients easily, if not too stressed
- clever, smart

Common Emotional issues

- fear/abandonment
- anger/shame
- cooperative, but may go to extreme of codependence
- orderly, but may be obsessive
- tends to bottle up anxiety until they explode
- tend to take things personally
- stressed nerves
- perfectionism

Physical Weaknesses

- physically sensitive
- mental stress
- sensitive digestive tract
- candida/fungus stress
- stress

Exercise

- rebounding
- resistance
- stretching
- isotonic exercises
- biking, swimming, hiking, dancing
- avoid heavy competitive sports

Weight Loss Tips

- avoid red meat as a Blood Type A stores meat as fat (needs to be modified if the person is a Metabolic Profile 2, as a #2 does not make purines in the body which are found in red meat)
- monitor food sources to eliminate fluid retention (often due to low stomach acid)
- avoid dairy as it impacts dairy reactions
- monitor wheat as it can increase acidity
- avoid kidney and lima beans as they slow metabolic rate
- pineapple and vegetables increase intestinal mobility
- soy foods can help improve digestion
- essential fatty acids (EFAs) help eliminate fluid retention and help with digestion

Common Diseases and Suggestions

Alcoholism
- often due to a lack of glyconutrients
- fungal imbalances

Anemia
- check for iron deficiency

Cancer
- anti-oxidants (monitor to prevent excess) such as quercetain and other phyto-chemicals
- green powders
- echinacea for the immune system
- colostrum
- glyconutrients

Candida
- most common problem of blood type As
- usually due to diet
- candida cleanse that has herbs to kill and probiotic support
- must follow a candida diet to eliminate Candida then follow with quality maintenance to avoid repeat

Colitis
- often due to wheat/dairy allergies
- probiotics
- enzymes

Heart Disease
- vitamin E
- coQ10
- garlic
- calcium and magnesium
- hawthorn

Liver and Gallbladder Disorders
- milk thistle
- liver cleanse

Type I Diabetes
- monitor diet, especially wheat and dairy
- support the pancreas
- chromium

Hormonal Imbalances
- wild yam capsules and/or creams
- soy
- alfalfa
- essential fatty acids (EFAs)

Parasites
- increase colostrum and probiotcs
- build immune system (glyconutrients)
- children's parasite cleanse

Pink Eye and Ear Infections in Children
- minimize or eliminate antibiotics
- build immune system (colostrum, glyconutrients, probiotcs)
- bifidus in children under the age of 6 instead of acidophilus

Thick Blood
- vitamins B, E
- essential fatty acids (EFAs)
- minerals (especially magnesium)

Stress
- chamomile as a herb or tea
- rescue remedy and/or other flower essences
- stress relieving homeopathics
- valerian as a herb or tea
- adrenal stress

Best Nutrients for Blood Type A
- cell essentials – smoothie
- minerals (magnesium, calcium, iron and zinc)
- chromium
- vitamins B, C and E
- wild yam
- cleanses (candida, parasite and liver)
- probiotics
- enzymes
- garlic
- lymph drainers
- colostsrum
- herbs (milk thistle, hawthorn, chamomile, echinacea, valerian)
- coQ10
- calming support

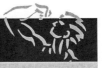

Blood Type B

The foods that have a "†" notation indicate foods that cause a high glycemic response. These foods should be omitted in order to lose fat.

If you have Candida, omit the foods that are *italicized* during a Candida cleanse. After the cleanse, or if you do not have Candida, use the foods accordingly.

Beneficial • Blood Type B

Proteins • Beneficial • Blood Type B

Meats

Lamb	Venison

Seafood

Cod	Mackerel	Salmon
Flounder	Mahi-mahi	Sea trout
Grouper	Ocean perch	Sole
Haddock	Pickerel	
Halibut	Pike	

Dairy and Eggs

Cottage cheese	*Goat cheese, milk*	*Mozzarella*
Farmer	*Kefir*	*Ricotta*
Feta	*Milk: skim, 2%*	*Yogurt: all*

Beans and Legumes

Kidney	Navy
Lima	Red

Fats • Beneficial • Blood Type B

Oils

Olive

Nuts and Seeds

None

Carbohydrates • Beneficial • Blood Type B

Cereals

Brown rice	*Oat: bran, oatmeal*
Millet	*Spelt*

Breads

Brown rice bread†	Millet†	*Sprouted bread: Alverado,*
Fin crisp†	Rice cakes†	*Essence, Ezekial, Manna*

Grains and Pastas
Flour: oat†, rice†

Vegetables • Beneficial • Blood Type B

Beets†	Collard greens	Parsnips†
Beet leaves	Eggplant	Peppers: green, jalapeno,
Broccoli	Kale	red, yellow
Brussels Sprouts	Lima beans	Sweet potatoes
Cabbage: all	Mushrooms: shitake	Yams: all
Carrots†	Mustard greens	
Cauliflower	Parsley	

Fruits • Beneficial • Blood Type B

Bananas	*Papaya*	*Plums: all*
Cranberries	*Grapes: all*	*Pineapple*

Juices • Beneficial • Blood Type B

Cabbage	*Grape*	*Pineapple*
Cranberry	*Papaya*	

Spices • Beneficial • Blood Type B

Cayenne pepper	Ginger	Parsley
Curry	Horseradish	

Condiments • Beneficial • Blood Type B

None

Herbs and Tea • Beneficial • Blood Type B

Ginger	Parsley	Rose hips
Ginseng	Peppermint	Sage
Licorice	Raspberry leaf	

Neutral Foods • Blood Type B

Proteins • Neutral • Blood Type B

Meats

Beef	Liver	Turkey
Buffalo	Pheasant	Veal

Seafood

Albacore (tuna)	Rainbow trout	White fish
Bluefish	Sailfish	
Herring	Snapper: all, red	

Seafood, continued

Perch: silver, yellow   Tilefish

Dairy and Eggs

Brie	Eggs	*Neufchatel*
Butter	*Edam*	*Parmesan*
Buttermilk	*Emmenthal*	*Provolone*
Camembert	*Gouda*	*Sherbet*
Casein	*Gruyere*	*Soy cheese, milk*
Cheddar	*Jarlsburg*	*Swiss*
Colby	*Monterey jack*	*Whey*
Cream cheese	*Munster*	*Whole milk*

Beans and Legumes

Broad†	Jicama	String
Cannellini	Northern	Tamarind
Copper	Peas: green, pods	White
Fava†	Red	
Green	Snap	

Fats • Neutral • Blood Type B

Oils

Flaxseed

Nuts and Seeds

Almonds, almond butter	Hickory	Pecans
Brazil nuts	Litchi	Walnuts
Chestnuts	Macadamia	

Carbohydrates • Neutral • Blood Type B

Cereals

Cream of rice†	Farina	Grape nuts†
Familia	Granola	

Breads

Gluten-free†	Oat bran muffins†	Soy
High-protein	Pumpernickel	*Spelt*

Grains and Pastas

Flour: graham†, *spelt*	Quinoa
Noodles: semolina, spinach	Brown rice: all

Vegetables • Neutral • Blood Type B

Aragula
Asparagus
Bamboo shoots
Bok choy
Celery
Chicory
Cucumber
Daikon radish
Dandelion
Endive
Escarole
Fennel
Garlic

Ginger
Horseradish
Kohlrabi
Leek
Lettuce: all
Mushrooms: all
Okra
Onions: all
Potatoes: all†
Radicchio
Rappini
Rutabaga
Scallions

Seaweed
Shallots
Snow peas
Spinach
Sprouts: alfalfa
Squash: all
Swiss chard
Turnips†
Water chestnut
Watercress
Zucchini

Fruits • Neutral • Blood Type B

Apples
Apricots†
Blackberries
Blueberries
Boysenberries
Cherries
Currants
Dates†
Elderberries
Figs

Gooseberries
Grapefruit
Guava
Kiwi
Kumquat
Lemons
Limes
Loganberries
Mangoes
Melon: all

Nectarines
Oranges
Peaches
Pears
Plantains
Prunes
Raisins
Raspberries
Strawberries
Tangerines

Juices • Neutral • Blood Type B

Apple
Apricot
Carrot†

Celery
Cherry: black
Cucumber

Grapefruit
Orange
Prune

Spices • Neutral • Blood Type B

Agar
Anise
Arrowroot
Basil
Bay leaf
Brown rice syrup†
Capers
Caraway
Cardamom
Carob

Dill
Dulse
Garlic
Honey†
Kelp
Maple syrup†
Marjoram
Mint
Miso
Mustard: dry

Pimento
Rosemary
Saffron
Sage
Salt: sea, Real™
Savory
Soy sauce
Spearmint
Sucanat†
Tamarind

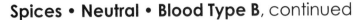
Spices • Neutral • Blood Type B, continued

Chervil
Chives
Chocolate
Cloves
Coriander
Cream of tartar
Cumin

Nutmeg
Oregano
Paprika
Parsley
Peppermint
Pepper: peppercorn,
  red flakes

Tarragon
Thyme
Turmeric
Vanilla
Vinegar: all
Wintergreen

Condiments • Neutral • Blood Type B

Apple butter
Mayonnaise

Mustard
Pickles: all

Relish
Worcestershire

Herbs and Tea • Neutral • Blood Type B

Alfalfa
Burdock
Catnip
Cayenne
Chamomile
Chickweed
Dandelion
Dong quai
Echinacea
Elder

Goldenseal
Green tea
Hawthorne
Horehound
Licorice root
Mulberry
St. John's wort
Sarsaparilla
Slippery elm
Spearmint

Strawberry leaf
Thyme
Valerian
Vervain
White birch
White oak bark
Yarrow
Yellow dock

Foods to Avoid • Blood Type B

Proteins • Avoid • Blood Type B

Meats

Chicken
Cornish hens
Duck

Goose
Partridge
Quail

Unclean meats

Seafood

Anchovy
Bluegill bass
Lox

Sea bass
Striped bass
Yellowtail

Unclean seafood

Dairy and Eggs

American cheese
Blue cheese

Ice cream
String cheese

Beans and Legumes

Aduke	Black-eyed peas	Lentils: all
Azuki	Garbanzo	
Black	Pinto	

Fats • Avoid • Blood Type B

Oils

Canola	Cottonseed	Sesame
Cashew	Peanut	Sunflower
Corn	Safflower	

Nuts and Seeds

Cashews	Pine nuts	Pumpkin seeds
Filberts	Pistachios	Sesame: butter, seeds
Peanuts: butter, nuts	Poppy seeds	Sunflower: butter, seeds

Carbohydrates • Avoid • Blood Type B

Cereals

Amaranth	Cream of wheat	Seven-grain
Barley	Kamut	Shredded wheat
Buckwheat	Kasha	Wheat: all
Corn: flakes, meal	Rye	

Breads

Bagels: wheat	Multi-grain bread	Wheat: all
Corn muffins	Rye bread: 100%	
Durum wheat	Rye: all	

Grains and Pastas

Buckwheat kasha	Pasta: artichoke	Wild rice
Couscous	Noodles: soba	
Flour: barley, bulghur, wheat, durum, gluten, rye		

Vegetable • Avoid • Blood Type B

Artichokes	Pumpkin	Tofu
Avocado	Radishes	Tomato
Corn: all	Sprouts: mung, radish	
Olives: all	Tempeh	

Fruits • Avoid • Blood Type B

Coconuts	Pomegranates	Rhubarb

Fruits • Avoid • Blood Type B, continued

Persimmons	Prickly pear	Starfruit

Juices • Avoid • Blood Type B

Tomato

Spices • Avoid • Blood Type B

Allspice	Cinnamon	Pepper: black ground, white
Almond extract	Corn: starch, syrup	Tapioca
Barley malt	Gelatin: plain	

Condiments • Avoid • Blood Type B

Ketchup

Herbs and Tea • Avoid • Blood Type B

Aloe	Hops	Senna
Coltsfoot	Linden	Shepherd's purse
Corn silk	Mullein	Skullcap
Fenugreek	Red clover	
Gentian	Rhubarb	

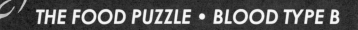

Blood Type B Summary Information

Strengths

- strong immune system
- adapts well to environmental conditions
- balanced nervous system
- sturdy and alert
- flexible
- less vulnerable to many diseases
- easy to work with other people

Common Emotional Issues

- anger/shame
- mercy
- over-extending themselves

Physical Weaknesses

- parasites
- brain stress
- auto-immune disorders such as lupus, multiple sclerosis and chronic fatigue
- dental issues and surgery stress

Exercise

- rebounding
- resistance
- hiking, cycling, tennis, swimming
- avoid extreme competitive exercises

Weight Loss Tips

- omit corn, lentils, peanuts and sesame seeds
- monitor blood sugar with enzymes and diet
- watch for poor assimilation of wheat, usually best to avoid for weight loss
- be sure to have green vegetables, especially salads
- protein and eggs usually increase metabolism

Common Diseases and Suggestions

Allergies (may have diarrhea)

- watch diet
- check for allergies
- enzymes (especially blood sugar balancing enzymes)

Brain Clarity

- ginkgo biloba
- lecithin

Chronic Fatigue

- adrenal support
- check diet
- immune support

Lou Gehrig's Disease

- mineral assimilation problems (Oligo mineral support can be helpful, also check pH)
- magnesium
- vitamin B
- colon cleanse

Lupus

- glyconutrients
- calcium and magnesium
- amino acids
- essential fatty acids (EFAs)

Multiple Sclerosis

- coQ10
- essential fatty acids (EFAs)
- garlic
- vitamin B
- colon cleanse

Best Nutrients for Blood Type B

- cell essentials – smoothie
- magnesium
- digestive enzymes
- ginkgo biloba
- lecithin
- adrenal support
- vitamin B
- colon cleanse

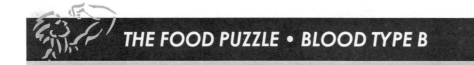

- glyconutrients
- garlic
- amino acids
- coQ10
- essential fatty acids (EFAs)

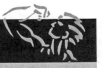

Blood Type AB

The foods that have a "†" notation indicate foods that cause a high glycemic response. These foods should be omitted in order to lose fat.

If you have Candida, omit the foods that are *italicized* during a Candida cleanse. After the cleanse, or if you do not have Candida, use the foods accordingly.

Beneficial • Blood Type AB

Proteins • Beneficial • Blood Type AB

Meats

Lamb	Turkey

Seafood

Albacore (tuna)	Snapper	Whitefish
Bluefish	Sole	
Perch: silver, white, yellow	Tilefish	

Dairy and Eggs

Cottage cheese	*Goat cheese, milk*	*Ricotta*
Farmer	*Kefir*	*Sour cream*
Feta	*Mozzarella*	*Yogurt: all*

Beans and Legumes

Lentils: green	Pinto	Red
Navy	Red soy	

Fats • Beneficial • Blood Type AB

Oils

Olive

Nuts and Seeds

Chestnuts	Peanuts, butter‡	Walnuts
‡Watch the mold content.		

Carbohydrates • Beneficial • Blood Type AB

Cereals

Millet†	Rice†
Oat bran, oatmeal	*Spelt*

Breads

100% Rye: bread, crisps†	Sprouted bread: *Alverado,*	Rice cakes†
Brown rice bread†	*Essene, Ezekial, Manna*	Soy flour bread
Fin crisp†	Millet†	

Grains and Pastas

Flour: oat†, rice†, rye†, *sprouted wheat*

Rice: basmati, brown, wild

Vegetables • Beneficial • Blood Type AB

Beets†	Cucumber	Parsnips†
Beet leaves	Eggplant	*Sweet potatoes*
Broccoli	Garlic	*Tempeh*
Cauliflower	Kale	*Tofu*
Celery	Mustard greens	*Yams: all*
Collard greens	Parsley	

Fruits • Beneficial • Blood Type AB

Cherries	Grapes: all	*Loganberries*
Cranberries	Grapefruit	*Pineapple*
Figs	*Kiwi*	*Plums*
Gooseberries	Lemons	

Juices • Beneficial • Blood Type AB

Cabbage	Cherry: black	Papaya
Carrot	Cranberry	
Celery	Grape	

Spices • Beneficial • Blood Type AB

Curry	Horseradish	Parsley
Garlic	*Miso*	

Condiments • Beneficial • Blood Type AB

None

Herbs and Tea • Beneficial • Blood Type AB

Alfalfa	Ginger	Licorice root
Burdock	Ginseng	Rose hips
Chamomile	Green tea	Strawberry leaf
Echinacea	Hawthorne	

Neutral • Blood Type AB

Proteins • Neutral • Blood Type AB

Meats

Liver	Pheasant

Seafood

Albacore (tuna)	Perch: silver, yellow, white	Sailfish
Bluefish	Rainbow trout	Tilefish
Herring (fresh)	Red snapper	Whitefish

Dairy and Eggs

Casein	*Emmenthal*	*Munster*
Cheddar	*Gouda*	*Neufchatel*
Colby	*Gruyere*	*Soy: all*
Cream cheese	*Jarlsburg*	*String*
Eggs	*Milk: 2%, skim*	*Swiss*
Edam	*Monterey jack*	*Whey*

Beans and Legumes

Broad†	Jicama	Snap
Cannellini	Lentils: domestic, red	String
Copper	Northern	Tamarind
Green beans	Peas: green, pods	White

Fats • Neutral • Blood Type AB

Oils

Canola	Flaxseed	Peanut oil

Nuts and Seeds

Almonds, butter	Hickory	Pine nuts
Brazil nuts	Litchi†	Pistachio
Cashews	Macadamia	

Carbohydrates • Neutral • Blood Type AB

Cereals

Amaranth	Farina	*Seven grain†*
Barley	*Cream of wheat†*	*Shredded wheat†*
Cream of rice†	*Granola*	Soy flakes: all
·Familia	*Grape nuts†*	*Wheat: bran, germ*

Breads

Bagels: wheat†	*Multi-grain†*	*Spelt*
Gluten-free†	Oat bran muffins†	*Wheat: durum†, whole bran*
High protein	Pumpernickel	
Matzos	Soy	

Grains and Pastas

Couscous	Flour: *durum†, spelt, wheat†*	Noodles: *spelt*, spinach
Flour: barley, bulgur	Noodles: semolina	Quinoa

Vegetables • Neutral • Blood Type AB

Arugula	Kohlrabi	Seaweed
Asparagus	Leek	Shallots
Bamboo shoots	Lettuce: all	Snow peas
Bok choy	*Mushrooms: domestic, enoki,*	Spinach
Cabbage: all	*oyster, portobello, tree*	Sprouts: Brussel
Carrots	Okra	Squash: all
Chicory	Olives: Greek, Spanish	Swiss chard
Daikon	Onions: all	Tomatoes
Dandelion	Potatoes: all†	Turnips
Endive	Pumpkin: all†	Water chestnut
Escarole	Radicchio	Watercress
Fennel	Rappini	Zucchini
Ginger	Rutabaga†	
Horseradish	Scallions	

Fruits • Neutral • Blood Type AB

Apples	*Elderberries*	*Pears*
Apricots	*Kumquat*	*Plantains*
Blackberries	*Limes*	*Prunes*
Blueberries	*Melons: all*	*Raisins*
Boysenberries	*Nectarines*	*Raspberries*
Currants	*Papayas*	*Strawberries*
Dates†	*Peaches*	*Tangerines*

Juices • Neutral • Blood Type AB

Apple	Cucumber	*Pineapple*
Apricot	*Grapefruit*	*Prune*

Spices • Neutral • Blood Type AB

Agar	Cumin	Saffron
Arrowroot	Dill	Sage
Basil	Dulse	Salt: sea, Real™
Bay leaf	*Honey†*	Savory
Brown rice syrup†	Kelp	*Soy sauce*
Cardamom	*Maple syrup†*	Spearmint
Carob	Marjoram	*Sucanat†*
Chervil	Mint	*Tamari*
Chives	Mustard: dry	Tamarind

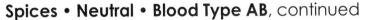

Spices • Neutral • Blood Type AB, continued

Chocolate	Nutmeg	Tarragon
Cinnamon	Paprika	Thyme
Cloves	Peppermint	Turmeric
Coriander	Pimento	Vanilla
Cream of tartar	Rosemary	Wintergreen

Condiments • Neutral • Blood Type AB

Mayonnaise	*Mustard*

Herbs and Tea • Neutral • Blood Type AB

Catnip	Mulberry	Spearmint
Cayenne	Parsley	Thyme
Chickweed	Peppermint	Valerian
Dandelion	Raspberry leaf	Vervain
Dong quai	Sage	White birch
Elder	Slippery elm	White oak bark
Goldenseal	St. John's wort	Yarrow
Horehound	Sarsaparilla	Yellow dock

Foods to Avoid • Blood Type AB

Proteins • Avoid • Blood Type AB

Meats

Beef	Duck	Quail
Buffalo	Goose	Veal
Chicken	Heart	Venison
Cornish hens	Partridge	

Seafood

Anchovy	Lox	Yellowtail
Bluegill bass	Sea bass	Unclean seafood
Halibut	Striped bass	

Dairy and Eggs

American cheese	Buttermilk	Parmesan
Blue cheese	Camembert	Provolone
Brie	Ice cream	Sherbet
Butter	Milk: whole	

Beans and Legumes

Aduke	Black-eyed peas	Kidney
Azuki	Fava	Lima

Beans and Legumes, continued

Black beans   Garbanzo

Fats • Avoid • Blood Type AB

Oils

Corn   Safflower   Sunflower
Cottonseed   Sesame

Nuts and Seeds

Filberts   Pumpkin seeds   Sunflower: seeds, butter
Poppy seeds   Sesame: seeds, butter

Carbohydrates • Avoid • Blood Type AB

Cereals

Buckwheat   Kamut
Corn: flakes, meal   Kasha

Breads

Corn muffins

Grains and Pastas

Buckwheat kasha   Pasta: artichoke   Noodles: soba

Vegetable • Avoid • Blood Type AB

Artichokes   Mushrooms: shitake   Radishes
Avocado   Olives: black   Sprouts: mung, radish
Corn: all   Peppers: green, jalapeno,
Lima beans   red, yellow

Fruits • Avoid • Blood Type AB

Bananas   Oranges   Rhubarb
Coconuts   Persimmons   Starfruit
Guava   Pomegranates
Mangoes   Prickly pear

Juices • Avoid • Blood Type AB

Orange

Spices • Avoid • Blood Type AB

Allspice   Capers   Tapioca
Almond extract   Corn: starch, syrup   Vinegar: all
Anise   Gelatin: plain
Barley malt   Pepper: all

Condiments • Avoid • Blood Type AB

Ketchup	Relish
Pickles: all	Worcestershire

Herbs and Tea • Avoid • Blood Type AB

Aloe	Hops	Senna
Coltsfoot	Linden	Shepherd's purse
Corn silk	Mullein	Skullcap
Fenugreek	Red clover	
Gentian	Rhubarb	

Blood Type AB Summary Information

Strengths

- all strengths of blood types A and B
- exhortation and encouragement
- spiritual strength
- popular
- charismatic

Common Emotional issues

- anger/shame
- resistance
- often ignores consequences of actions
- often appear disloyal
- hurtful to others

Physical Weaknesses

- hormonal imbalances
- sensitive digestive system
- candida and parasites
- immune sensitivity

Exercise

- rebounding
- resistance
- hiking, cycling, tennis, swimming

Weight Loss Tips

- avoid red meat and chicken
- don't skip meals and be sure to eat a good breakfast
- avoid carbonated beverages as they reduce gastrin production which can inhibit digestion
- monitor food combinations and whether digestive enzymes are helpful to ensure proper digestion of food (best food combination tip is to avoid protein and starch consumption at the same meal)

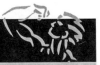
Common Diseases and Suggestions

Anemia

- iron
- blood cleansers such as red clover

Cancer, Especially Breast Cancer

- glyconutrients
- wild yam
- coQ10
- garlic
- vitamin C
- echinacea

Digestion

- low stomach acid (need HCl)
- enzymes

Gallbladder Stress

- avoid nuts, use nut butters
- enzymes, especially fat-digesting enzymes
- liver cleanse

Heart Disease

- vitamin E
- minerals, especially magnesium
- colon cleanse
- liver cleanse
- hawthorn

PMS, Menopause Problems

- wild yam
- soy
- alfalfa
- avoid HRT (hormone replacement therapy in synthetic form)

Thick Mucus/Blood

- mucus drainers
- lemon in pure water daily
- avoid allergenic foods
- colon cleanse

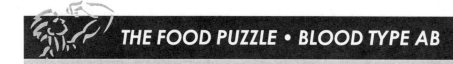

Best Nutrients for Blood Type AB

- cell essentials – smoothie
- glyconutrients
- vitamin C
- vitamin E
- wild yam
- herbs (such as alfalfa, red clover, hawthorn, echinacea, milk thistle)
- mucus drainers
- enzymes, HCl, bromelain
- colon cleanse
- iron
- magnesium
- coQ10
- garlic
- rescue remedy
- calming herbs (such as valerian root and chamomile)

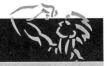

RECOMMENDED BRANDS

Recommended Brands for Nutrient Sources for all Blood Types

Overview

Many people take many supplements, often with no plan or purpose other than to address symptoms. Cell Essentials is more than just a phrase; it is an approach to health based on building healthy cells. The nutrients in the Cell Essentials, along with rebounding (we like to call it Cellercise) are key to building healthy cells and the foundation for any good supplement program.

The following overview will help you understand the need for each of the key categories. The first three categories, Essential Amino Acids, Essential Fatty Acids, and Essential Carbohydrates are essential; they are the basic building blocks for healthy cells.

Cell Essentials

Essential Amino Acids (Protein Powder)

Amino acids are the building blocks of protein. Providing the cells with essential amino acids from non-meat sources provides the benefits of protein without the negatives of excess animal protein. Protein supplies the amino acids your body needs to support the growth of all blood cells, muscles and other tissues. In addition, protein is needed to produce hormones such as insulin, antibodies to fight disease and the enzymes that are essential for digestion.

Protein powders made without soy are better for blood types O and B. Be sure to read the label, as the ratio of protein, carbohydrates and sugars will vary significantly. You want a high protein with low sugar and low carbohydrate levels. The brands listed below have tested well.

Essential Fatty Acids (Flaxseed Oil)

Essential fatty acids are considered essential nutrients in that the body cannot make them. All cells in the body are enveloped by a membrane composed mainly of essential fatty acids called phospholipids. These lipids are key in determining cell integrity and fluidity. A deficiency of these lipids makes it virtually impossible for the cell membranes to perform vital functions such as regulation of what goes in/out of the cell, maintaining homeostasis and virtually all other cellular functions.

Evening primrose oil, black currant seed oil and borage oil are high in omega-6 fatty acids. Fish oils and flaxseed oil are rich in omega-3 fatty acids. Research indicates the ratio between the two should be 4 (Omega-6) to 1 (Omega-3). Most Americans get ten to twenty times the amount of Omega 6 fatty acids (low quality grocery store oils and processed foods). This imbalance is responsible for many of the health problems we see today. As a result, it is essential for most Americans to supplement their intake of omega-3.

Omega-3 fatty acids are known to help lower cholesterol and blood pressure, reduce allergic and inflammatory conditions, reduce MS symptoms and help fight cancer. Many other benefits are known to occur from the intake of omega-3 fatty acids, including: weight loss, improved skin quality, reduction of cysts, reduced risk of diabetes, improved immune disorders, reduced hormonal imbalances, improved vision and a healthier pregnancy.

My experience with over 2,000 clinical tests has shown no other omega-3 oil has surpassed Barlean's High Lignan Flaxseed Oil in quality and bio-availability.

Essential Carbohydrates (Glyconutrients)

To maintain a healthy body, cells must "talk" to other cells. Their "language" is one of touch written in saccharides on cell membranes. These simple sugars (not table sugar!) combine with other molecules to make glycoforms. An example would be combining saccharides with amino acids to form glycoproteins or saccharides combined with lipids to form glycolipids. Of the 200 monosaccharides (single sugars) that occur naturally in plants, eight have been discovered to be essential glycoforms (cell communicators). Like thousands of different "keys" projecting from the cell surface, they will either "unlock" the required functions of the adjoining cell or not. If the right keys are available, the body functions smoothly. If not, it doesn't. This lack of proper "cell to cell" communication is seen manifested in many of the "new" autoimmune diseases that were rare just 30 – 40 years ago and today are considered common and normal.

Of those eight saccharides only two are found in our processed, refined food diets. We are no longer eating the foods that naturally supplied these essential sugars. While the body has the ability to manufacture all of these eight saccharides, it requires a complicated conversion process that requires numerous enzymes and vitamins. People who are ill, or have inborn errors of metabolism are especially vulnerable to breakdown in that conversion process. Whenever these necessary monosaccharides cannot be made, cellular communication is slowed or impaired. The only source for all eight saccharides in a single nutritional supplement is Ambrotose by Mannatech.

When we have a deficiency of any of these three cell essentials, essential amino acids, essential fatty acids, and essential carbohydrates, it is impossible for the body to maintain a state of optimal health. As it works to compensate for these deficiencies, cellular, organ and tissue stress occurs and we have begun the disease process. In today's world of processed, packaged, fast foods, it is impossible to get all of these essentials without supplementation!

Cell Essentials (take in your daily smoothie drink)

Category	Preferred Brand(s)
Amino acids (protein powder)	Bio-Phase, Natren, Designer Protein, NutriBiotic
Flax oil	Barlean's High Lignan Flaxseed Oil
Glyconutrients	Ambrotose by Mannatech

Cell Beneficials

There are three other nutrients that are highly beneficial for your cells. Although they are not part of the essential three, they are key for optimal immune function.

Colostrum

Colostrum is the first mammary secretion that every mammal gives its newborn. It contains numerous compounds that affect more than fifty processes in the body, ranging from immunity to regeneration and growth of all types of cells.

The immune and growth factors contained in bovine (cow) colostrum have been shown to be identical to those found in human colostrum – not just identical, but many times more potent. The

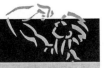

immune factors in colostrum contain antibodies that provide immunity from numerous microorganisms.

The growth factors in colostrum are responsible for the rebuilding and repair of cellular tissues. They improve nutrient intake, rebuild bone mass, return elasticity to the skin, improve energy, build lean muscle, increase memory, balance blood sugar levels, burn fat and elevate moods. Check the following for brand recommendations.

Ionic Minerals

In today's world, naturally occurring nutrient-rich soil is becoming more and more rare. Many of the trace elements once abundant in soil have been washed into the oceans. In oceans they are found in their proper proportions – the same found in healthy human bodies.

Minerals are needed for every electrical function in the body. Every second of every day your body relies on ionic minerals (charged minerals for quick absorption) and trace minerals to conduct and generate billions of tiny electrical impulses. Without these impulses, not a single muscle, including the heart, would be able to function. The brain would not function and cells would not be able to use osmosis to balance water pressure and absorb nutrients.

Minerals are of no value if they cannot be absorbed. Mineral absorption primarily takes place in the small intestine. As food matter passes through the intestines, minerals transfer into the blood stream through the walls of the intestines. This can only happen if the minerals are ionically charged. Although stomach acid helps ionize the minerals in foods, an ionized mineral supplement supports this process.

Trace minerals exist in a synergistic relationship to each other. Taking too much of one can imbalance others. Taking an ionized, synergistic blend of minerals increases absorption and decreases the possibility of a mineral imbalance. See below for brand recommendation.

Green Powders

Life on earth would be impossible without chlorophyll, one of the key nutrients in green foods. Chlorophyll is key for cleansing and building the blood as well as detoxifying the liver.

Green powders are the condensed forms of rich, green foods. The common sources of these green powders are cereal grasses such as kamut, wheat, barley, oats and alfalfa; blue-green algae species such as spirulina and chlorella; and dark green land and sea vegetables.

Green drinks can be made at home by juicing fresh grasses. However, for most people that is too time-consuming. The following brands are good sources of green powders, an easy addition to the LFH smoothie.

Cell Beneficials (additional support for your smoothie)

Category	Preferred Brand(s)
Colostrum	Immune-Tree, ImmunoStart by Mannatech
Ionic liquid minerals	Concentrace Mineral Drops Trace Minerals
Greens	Barlean's Greens, KyoGreen by Kyolic, PhytAloe by Mannatech

Other Key Supplemental Support

Multi-Vitamin/Mineral and Individual Vitamin Support

Category	Preferred Brand(s)
Multi-Vitamin/Min	Catalyst by Mannatech
Kids Multi-Vitamin/Min	GlycoBEARS by Mannatech
B	Standard Process Cataplex B, Cataplex G
C	Manna C from Mannatech and Enzyme Solution #3
E	Unique E by AC Grace
CoQ10	Standard Process
Calcium	
If pH is acid	CO by Nutritional Resources
	Alkazyme by Apex
If pH is alkaline	CL by Nutritional Resources
General	Cal Zyme by Apex
	Cal/Mag by Trace Minerals

Enzymes – for a customized enzyme protocol complete the LFH Enzyme Questionnaire.

Category	Preferred Brand(s)
Protease/protein enzymes	Enzyme Solutions #11
Carbohydrate assimilation	Enzyme Solutions #14
HCL	ZymeMAX by Advanced Nutritionals
	Enzyme Solutions #12

Probiotics – healthy bacteria for intestinal trace

Category	Preferred Brand(s)
L. Acidophilus	FloraMAX by Advanced Nutritionals, Kyodophilus by Kyolic or Megadophilus by Natren
B. Bifidum	FloraMAX by Advanced Nutritionals, Kyodophilus by Kyolic, Bifido by Natren

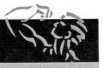
Hormone Support – for healthy male and female hormones

Category	Preferred Brand(s)
Wild yam	Plus by Mannatech, Enzyme Solutions #23
Wild yam creams	Fem-Gest by Bio Nutritional Formulas
Saw palmetto for men	Enzyme Solutions #22

Herbs

For individual or herbal blends I recommend Nature's Sunshine

Flower therapies – for emotional support

Category	Preferred Brand(s)
Individual and flower blends	Ellon and Bach Flower Essences
Rescue remedy	Calming Essence by Ellon, Rescue Remedy by Bach

Lymph and Drainage Support – for clearing toxins

This should be recommended by your health care provider or by a LFH Coach based on case history.

Rebounding, call the LFH office for a free "phone class" on this great form of exercise.

Skin brushing, *Skin Brushing the Gaither Way*, a video, and skin brushes available from LFH.

Cleanses

To be done twice a year or under the direction of your health care provider or LFH Coach.

Category	Preferred Brand(s)
Parasite	ParaMAX by Advanced Naturals
Liver	Liver Detox by Advanced Naturals
Heavy Metals	Heavy Metal Detox by Advanced Naturals
General detoxification	CleanseMAX by Advanced Naturals
Colon cleanse	ColonMAX by Advanced Naturals

Other

Adrenal Support – needed during times of added stress.

Category	Preferred Brand(s)
Adrenal support	Enzyme Solutions #13, Adrenal Terrain by Apex

Recommended Brands for Candida Cleansing

Category	Preferred Brand(s)
General Cleanse	CandiMAX by Advanced Naturals
Homeopathic Cleanse	LVR/DRN and YST/CAN by Apex Fungi Fuge by Genex
Children's Cleanse	ParaGONE by Advanced Naturals (pills) Fungi Fuge by Genex (liquid)
Heavy Metal Cleanse	Heavy Metal Cleanse by Advanced Naturals
Probiotic	FloraMAX by Advanced Naturals Kyodophilus by Kyolic Megadophilus and Bifido by Natren Enzyme Solutions #17
Enzymes	Enzyme Solutions (based on your enzyme questionnaire)
Fiber	FiberMAX by Advanced Naturals
Garlic	Kyolic Aged Garlic
Stevia	Stevia Clear by Wisdom of the Ancients
Adrenal Support	Enzyme Solutions Formula 13 (capsule) Adrenal Terrain by APEX (liquid) DSF by Nutri-West (glandular support)

Recommended Brands for Equipment

Juicer	Champion Juicer

TESTS

Stomach Acid Test

15 – 20 minutes after eating a meal, drink the following mixture
- 1 tablespoon of cider vinegar
- mixed with 2 tablespoons of pure water

One of two things will happen:
- feel better, which is an indication of low stomach acid (HCl support is needed)
- feel worse (less common), which is an indication of excess stomach acid (DGL and/or alkaline support is needed)

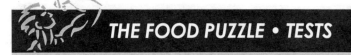

Allergy Test

A simple way to determine if a food is allergenic is to use the following test:
1. Take resting pulse rate (heart beats per minute)
2. Eat suspected food in its simplest form (i.e., corn vs. vegetable soup)
3. Wait 20 minutes
4. Retake resting pulse rate.

If the second pulse rate is 10+ points higher, then avoid the food.
If the second pulse rate is the same or only a few points higher, the food is not stressing the body.

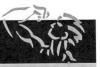

Enzyme Questionaire

Metabolic enzymes are needed for every function in the body. This questionnaire identifies the top metabolic functions that are being hindered by a lack of enzymes.

Please score each question as follows:

3 = if this is a MAJOR problem
1 = if this is a MINOR problem

(If you never have the problem leave it blank)

Group 1
1. Would you describe yourself as a Type A personality, for example – driven or aggressive? _____
2. Tendency to problems of indigestion or constipation _____
3. Stiff joints, especially after rest, i.e., loss of mobility _____
4. Sensitive to sudden sounds, i.e., startle easily __1__
5. Headaches in back of head and neck _____
6. Spacey and forgetful _____
7. Flutters in your (heart) chest __1__

subtotal _____

Group 2
1. History of diabetes _____
2. High blood pressure _____
3. High blood triglyceride levels _____
4. Dizziness or light-headedness when changing positions _____
5. Headaches on side of the head and temples _____

subtotal _____

Group 3
1. History of cataracts, glaucoma or poor vision _____
2. Frequent head colds, runny nose and/or watery eyes _____
3. Bruise easily and/or slow healing of cuts, sore or bleeding gums, gingivitis _____
4. Frequent headaches associated with eyestrain or pain upon moving eyes _____
5. Frequent redness in the eyelids or "sand in your eyes" _____
6. Exposure to toxins and chemicals _____

subtotal _____

Group 4

1. History of chronic sinus problems
2. Loss of sense of smell, or an obstruction to nasal breathing
3. Bothered by thick mucous in sinuses or discharge from nose
4. Frequent nosebleeds
5. Facial pain or paralysis

subtotal

Group 5

1. Histories of spinal disc problems or back surgery
2. Cannot tolerate stress, i.e., unable to make decisions — 1
3. Irritated or receding gums, loose teeth
4. Cold hands and feet — 3
5. Clicking jaw or jaw pain

subtotal

Group 6

1. History of speech impediment, stuttering or stammering
2. Dry, itchy eyes, or dry mouth
3. Poor memory — 1
4. Inability to relax, become serene or meditate — 1
5. Frequent sore throat, or sores on tongue or in mouth
6. Tendency for swollen glands
7. Cold or canker sores

subtotal

Group 7

1. History of thyroid gland disorders or medication
2. Fast heartbeat, i.e., racing heart
3. Swollen or painful breasts
4. Moist warm skin, i.e., sweat easily
5. Neck, shoulder, arm or hand pain

subtotal

Group 8

1. History of frequent canker sores, cold blisters or boils
2. Muscle and tendon weakness, pain in low back and buttocks
3. Slow morning starter, writer's cramp or stiffness after sitting
4. Dry skin, dandruff, hair falling out
5. Painful ribs, pleurisy, pain on inhalation, or sharp chest or shoulder pain

subtotal

Group 9
1. History of heart disease, taking medications, etc. ____
2. Irregular heartbeat or skipped beats _1_
3. Dryness of skin and hair, itching due to dryness ____
4. Have varicose veins and/or hemorrhoids ____
5. Shoulder or chest pain on exertion ____

subtotal ____

Group 10
1. History of asthma, emphysema, bronchitis or pneumonia ____
2. Difficulty breathing, shortness of breath ____
3. Frequent cough, dry or productive ____
4. Wheezing or difficulty breathing when lying on back ____
5. Shoulder pain or bursitis ____

subtotal ____

Group 11
1. History of gall bladder stones or surgery ____
2. Loss of appetite, especially for meat ____
3. Frequent sour taste in mouth, intolerance of fats and spicy foods ____
4. Have frequent constipation with light colored stools ____
5. Discomfort or soreness under the right rib cage after eating ____

subtotal ____

Group 12
1. History of ulcers or gastritis ____
2. Frequent heartburn or indigestion with nausea and pain ____
3. Acid reflux after eating ____
4. Frequent use of antacids ____
5. Pain or burning in the stomach that is relieved by eating ____

subtotal ____

Group 13
1. History of low blood pressure problems ____
2. Awake after a few hours of rest and cannot go back to sleep _1_
3. Suffer from frequent periods of depression or inability to think clearly ____
4. Become light-headed when meals are missed ____
5. Suffer from frequent nightmares or panic attacks ____
6. Periods of exhaustion after stress ____

subtotal ____

Group 14

1. History of lactose intolerance or gluten intolerance
2. Craving or thirst for cold liquids or foods _____
3. Intolerance of dairy products, grains or sugar _____
4. Sensitive to air pollutants, such as perfumes, smoke, etc. _____
5. Discomfort or soreness under the left rib cage after eating _____
6. Heartburn after eating _____

subtotal _____

Group 15

1. History of anemia or other blood disorder, or taking medication _____
2. Fatigue, tired most of the time _____
3. Pale skin, lips and nails _____
4. Low resistance (frequent colds and infections) _____
5. Getting sleepy after eating _____
6. FEMALES: undo fatigue after menstrual flow _7_

subtotal _____

Group 16

1. History of hepatitis, jaundice or other liver disorder _____
2. History of high blood pressure and/or medication _____
3. Water retention, swelling of hands and feet _____
4. Varicose veins and/or hemorrhoids _____
5. Shoulder and neck stiffness and/or soreness _____

subtotal _____

Group 17

1. History of chronic or frequent yeast infections _____
2. Foul odor to stool and urine _____
3. Unusually large appetite, i.e., cannot control the urge to eat _____
4. Frequent or prolonged use of antibiotics _____
5. Constipation with hard, dry stool _____
6. Athlete's foot, crumbly toenails _____

subtotal _____

Group 18

1. History of reactive hypoglycemia _____
2. Suffer from airborne allergies _____
3. Dark circles under the eyes _____
4. Nausea or vomiting type of indigestion or morning sickness _____
5. Muscular low back pain _____

subtotal _____

Group 19

1. History of skin disorders, such as acne
2. Dermatitis, eczema or psoriasis $\frac{1}{3}$
3. Have many warts and moles
4. Frequent episodes of hives due to food allergies
5. Excessive perspiration or lack of perspiration

           subtotal _____

Group 20

1. History of constipation with infrequent bowel movements
2. Frequent use of laxatives or enemas
3. Hard, painful stools
4. Lower abdominal gas
5. Less than one bowel movement a day
6. Pain in right lower abdomen

           subtotal _____

Group 21

1. History of colitis or other disease of the large intestine
2. Diarrhea with mucous or blood in stool
3. Frequent or soft bowel movements
4. Lower left bowel pain
5. Painful bowel movements

           subtotal _____

Group 22

1. History of prostate disorders or medication
2. Frequent night urination
3. Dribbling
4. Loss of sexual urge   3
5. Pain radiating into the groin or testes

           subtotal _____

Group 23

1. History of hysterectomy or estrogen replacement therapy
2. Vaginal discharge
3. Excessive menstrual flow
4. Lack of menstruation, scanty flow or irregular period
5. Painful periods and/or symptoms of PMS   1

           subtotal _____

Group 24
1. History of frequent bladder infections   _____
2. Frequent urination, urgency or loss of control   _____
3. Pass small amounts of urine at each voiding   _____
4. Dry skin, flaking and dandruff   _____
5. Pain or discomfort over the bladder   _____

subtotal   _____

Group 25
1. History of bone disorders, spurs, osteoporosis, etc.   _____
2. Muscle soreness and weakness   _____
3. Painful or loose teeth or poor fitting dentures   _____
4. Hyper-irritability, insomnia, and/or restlessness   _____
5. Low back pain, weak joints or ligaments, fallen arches   _____
6. Weak, ridged or split fingernails   _____

subtotal   _____

Group 26
1. History of injury to the tailbone   _____
2. Restlessness or insomnia   _____
3. Inability to concentrate, frequent day-dreaming or nightmares   _____
4. Unresolved health problems   _____
5. Painful tailbone, i.e., hurts to sit down   _____
6. History of sexual, physical or emotional abuse   1

subtotal   _____

Group 27
1. History of muscle soreness and pain after exercise   _____
2. Inability to tolerate potassium-rich foods such as molasses or olives   _____
3. Frequent writer's cramp or stiffness especially after rest   _____
4. Muscle soreness and pain resulting from exercise   _____
5. Loss of joint range of motion, painful stretching   _____
6. Allergies, hay fever, hives   _____
7. Rashes, psoriasis, eczema or other skin problems   1

subtotal   _____

Group 28
1. History of deep bone or joint pain, painful weak teeth   _____
2. Frequent anxiety, use of tranquilizers   _____
3. Frequent infections, need for antibiotics   _____
4. Symptoms of edema, such as swelling of feet and ankles   _____
5. Recent acute traumatic incidents or accidents   _____

subtotal   _____

Group 29
1. Always tired, i.e., unable to meet daily requirements   _____
2. Loss of appetite or feel better if you don't eat   _____
3. Restless sleep, gnawing of teeth   _____
4. Thin and have difficulty gaining weight   _____
5. Itching around rectum and groin   _____

                                                            subtotal _____

Group 30
1. History of chronic indigestion   _____
2. Unusual fullness after eating   _____
3. Lower bowel gas   _____
4. Undigested food, capsules or tablets found in the stool   _____
5. Frequent abdominal cramping after eating   _____

                                                            subtotal _____

Group 31
1. Generalized malaise, i.e., lackadaisical attitude   _____
2. Frequent lack of motivation, unable to get started   _____
3. Fatigued, easily tired   _____
4. Failure to meet ordinary requirements of daily activities   _____
5. Failure to respond to specific nutritional schedules   _____

                                                            subtotal _____

Group 32
1. History of pernicious anemia   _____
2. Loss of taste for meat   _____
3. Strong desire to eat when not hungry   _____
4. Indigestion, particularly 2 to 3 hours after eating   _____
5. Flatulence, lower bowel gas   _____

                                                            subtotal _____

Group 33
1. History of diabetes in your family   _____
2. Blood sugar problems, either hypoglycemia or diabetes   _____
3. Unable to control appetite   _____
4. Desire to lose weight   _____
5. Need a meal replacement   _____

                                                            subtotal _____

Group 34
1. Painful gas
2. Bloating after eating dairy   _____
3. Diarrhea after eating dairy   _____
                                                                  _____

                                                    subtotal   _____

Group 35
1. History of osteoarthritis or gout
2. Musculoskeletal pain, difficulty walking, etc.   _____
3. Bone and joint pain in spine, hips, knees, feet or hands   _____
4. Inflammation, i.e., fever, redness, swelling and/or pain   _____
5. Stiff joints, sore muscles or diagnosed with fibromyalgia   _____
                                                                  _____

                                                    subtotal   _____

Group 36
1. History of chronic herpes-type skin eruptions, such as frequent canker sores,
    cold blisters and boils   _____
2. Raised and red skin eruptions such as hives, strong reaction to food or chemicals   _____
3. Strong reactions to mosquito or insect bites   _____
4. Frequent histamine reactions, such as sneezing attacks, etc. _____
5. Painful skin irritations such as sunburn, diaper rash or chapped lips   _____

                                                    subtotal   _____

Group 1 correlates with Enzyme 1, Group 2 – Enzyme 2 and so on. The group that has the highest match to your symptoms is the enzyme you would need. *Up to three different enzymes can be taken without scheduling a consultation. (Be sure to note when enzymes are to be taken for maximum results.)*

SMOOTHIE RECIPE

Ingredients

- 1 – 1½ cups liquid (water, almond milk, rice milk, soy milk or fruit juice†)
- ½ banana (optional based on blood type)
- ¼ – ½ cup fresh or frozen fruit (based on blood type)
- ice
- Cell Essentials™
- optional additions

Directions

Blend in blender.

Makes 1 smoothie for an adult (enough for 2 children). During travel, the basic smoothie can be placed in a shaker and shook.

† almond milk is lower on the glycemic index than rice or soy milk or fruit juice

Cell Essentials™

- 1 – 2 scoops of protein powder
  (1 scoop for Profile 1, 1½ scoops for Profile 2, 2 scoops for Profile 3)
  recommendations can be found in the Recommended Brands Chapter
- 1 – 2 Tablespoon of flaxseed oil
  (1 tablespoon for Profile 1, 1½ tablespoons for Profile 2, 2 tablespoons for Profile 3)
  recommend Barlean's Flaxseed oil
- ¼ – ½ teaspoons of glyconutrients
  recommend Ambrotose™ by Mannatech

Optional Ingredients

- 10 – 20 drops of Trace Minerals ConcenTrace Drops
- 1 – 3 teaspoons of a green powder
- 1 teaspoon of colostrum
  recommendations can be found in the Recommended Brands Chapter

Note

Change the liquid source and fruits for variety and flavor. Learn to make a smoothie in such a way that you enjoy it. It can be delicious and great for you!

BIBLIOGRAPHY

Bach, Edward, M.D., *Heal Thyself*, Reproduced by Keats Publishing, 1931.

Ballentine, Rudolph M.D., *Diet and Nutrition — A Holistic Approach*, Himalayan International Institute, Honesdale, PA, 1978.

Berquist, Maurice, *The Miracle and Power of Blessing*, Warner Press, Inc, Anderson, IN, 1983.

Biermann, June and Barbara Toohey, *The Diabetics Total Health Book*, Tarcher Putnam, NY, NY, 1992.

Brand, Dr. Paul and Philip Yancey, *Fearfully and Wonderfully Made*, Zondervan Publishing House, Grand Rapids, MI, 1980.

Carter, Albert E., *The New Miracles of Rebound Exercise*, A.L.M. Publishers, Fountain Hills, AZ, 1988.

Cook, Trevor M., Ph.D., *A Beginner's Introduction for Homeopathy*, Keats Publishing, Inc., New Canaan, CT, 1987.

Cummings, Stephen., M.D., and Dana Ullman, M.P.H., *Everybody's Guide to Homeopathic Medicines*, Jeremy P. Tarcher/Putnam, NY, NY, 1997.

D'Adamo, Dr. Peter J., with Catherine Whitney, *Eat Right For Your Blood Type*, G.P. Putnam's Sons, NY, NY, 1997.

D'Adamo, Peter J. N.D., *Live Right For Your Type*, G.P. Putnam's Sons, NY, NY, 2001.

DuBelle, Lee, *Proper Food Combining Works — Living Testimony*, Lee DuBelle, Phoenix, AZ, 1997.

Fife, Bruce, N.D., *The Detox Book, HealthWise*, Colorado Springs, CO, 1997.

Fitzgerald, Patricia, C.N., *The Detox Solution*, Illumination Press, Santa Monica, 2001.

Frähm, Dave, *A Cancer Battle Plan Sourcebook*, Jeremy P. Tarcher/Putnam, NY, NY, 2000.

Frähm, Dave, *Healthy Habits*, Piñon Press, Colorado Springs, CO, 1993.

Gebauer, Ray, *How to Cure and Prevent any Disease*, Freedom Unlimited, Inc., Bellevue, WA, 2000.

Gerber, Richard, M.D., *Vibrational Medicine*, Bear & Company, Santa Fe, NM, 1996.

Gittleman, Ann Louise, M.S.: *Your Body Knows Best*, Pocket Books, NY, NY, 1997.

Kersey, Cynthia, *Unstoppable*, Sourcebooks, Inc., Naperville, IL, 1998.

Kirban, Salem, *How to Eat Your Way Back to Vibrant Health*, Salem Kirban, Inc., Huntingdon Valley, PA, 1977.

Levy, Susan L., D.C. and Carol Lehr, M.A., *Your Body Can Talk*, Hohm Press, Prescott, AZ, 1996.

McGee, Robert S. and Donald W. Sapaugh, *The Search for Peace*, Servant Publications, Ann Arbor, MI, 1996.

Miller, Jennie Ph.D., Johanna Burani, M.S., R. D., C.D.E., Kaye Foster-Powell, B.Sc., M. Nutri. & Diet, *The Glucose Revolution Life Plan,* Marlowe & Company, NY, NY, 2001.

Morter, Dr. M. Ted, Jr., M.A., *Your Health ... Your Choice*, Lifetime Books, Inc., Hollywood, FL, 1998.

Murray, Michael T. N.D., and Jade Beutler, R.R.T., R.C.P, *Understanding Fats & Oils,* PHP Publishing, Encinitas, CA, 1996.

Murray, Michael, T. N.D., *Diabetics and Hypoglycemia,* Prima Publishing, Rocklin, CA, 1994.

Pederson, Mark, *Nutritional Herbology — A Reference Guide to Herbs*, Wendell W. Whitman Company, Warsaw, IN, 1998.

Russel, Rex, M.D., *What the Bible Says About Healthy Living*, Regal Books, Ventura, CA, 1996.

Steward, H. Leighton, M.S., Morrison C. Bethea, M.D., Sam S. Andrews, M.D., Luis A. Balart, M.D., *Sugar Busters*, Ballantine Books, NY, NY, 1998.

Tessler, Gordon S., Ph.D. and Laura Tessler, *Cooking For Life*, Be Well Publications, Raleigh, NC, 1995.

Tessler, Gordon S., Ph.D., *The Genesis Diet*, Be Well Publications, Raleigh, NC, 1996.

Townsley, Cheryl, *Candida Made Simple*, LFH Publications, Littleton, CO, 1997.

Townsley, Cheryl, *Cleansing Made Simple*, rev. ed., LFH Publications, Littleton, CO, 2001.

Townsley, Cheryl, *Discovering Wholeness*, LFH Publications, Littleton, CO, 2000.

Townsley, Cheryl, *Food Smart!*, Jeremy P. Tarcher/Putnam, NY, NY, 1999.

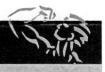

Townsley, Cheryl, *Kid Smart!*, LFH Publications, Littleton, CO, 1998.

Townsley, Cheryl, *Lifestyle for Health Cookbook*, LFH Publications, Littleton, CO, 1995.

Townsley, Cheryl, *Meals in 30 Minutes*, rev. ed., Littleton, CO: LFH Publications, 1997.

Truman, Karol K., *Feelings Buried Alive Never Die ...*, Olympus Distributing, Las Vegas, NV, 1991.

Williams, Dr. Roger J., *The Wonderful World Within You*, Bio-Communications Press, Wichita, KS, 1977.

Wright, Pastor Henry, *A More Excellent Way*, Pleasant Valley Publications, Thomaston, GA, 1999.

Zand, Jane, Lac, OMD and Rachel Walton, RN and Bob Roundtree, M.D., *Smart Medicine for a Healthier Child*, Avery Publishing Group, Garden City Park, NY, 1994.

THE AUTHOR

Dr. Cheryl Townsley is a Naturopathic Doctor, Master Herbalist and advanced graduate of the International Academy of Bioelectric Practitioners. She also holds degrees in home economics and computer science.

Dr. Townsley is the founder of Lifestyle for Health, a company dedicated to helping people restore their wholeness in order to live out their God-given potential. In pursuit of that goal, she has lectured internationally and been featured on hundreds of national and international television and radio shows. She trains practitioners on their understanding of emotional contributions to physical sickness and disease.

Dr. Townsley directs a successful wellness clinic that helps people identify the key stressors in their life and build a customized protocol for wellness. In addition to working with clients, Cheryl has authored eleven books and an international newsletter.

Cheryl Townsley resides in Denver, Colorado, with her husband Forest and their daughter, Anna.

Lifestyle for Health Order Form

		Quantity	Total

Books

Discovering Wholeness, Townsley	26.95	_____	_____
Food Smart!, Townsley	13.00	_____	_____
Kid Smart!, Townsley	15.00	_____	_____
Cleansing Made Simple, Townsley	10.00	_____	_____
Candida Simple, Townsley	12.00	_____	_____
Return to Paradise, Townsley	10.00	_____	_____
Healthy Habits, Frähm	13.00	_____	_____

Cookbooks

Lifestyle for Health Cookbook, Townsley	26.00	_____	_____
Meals in 30 Minutes, Townsley	15.00	_____	_____
Candida Control Cookbook, Burton	14.00	_____	_____
Stevia Sweet Recipes, Goettemoeller	13.95	_____	_____

Audio Education

Too Stressed to Be Blessed (4 tapes)	25.00	_____	_____
Raging Hormones (4 tapes)	25.00	_____	_____
Healthy Kids – Beating ADD (2 tapes)	15.00	_____	_____
Supplements – A Systems Approach (1 tape)	5.00	_____	_____
Health & Supplements on a Budget (1 tape)	5.00	_____	_____
Top 10 Health Builders & Busters (2 tapes w/notes)	20.00	_____	_____
Optimal Health Video	25.00	_____	_____
Skin Brushing the Gaither Way	30.00	_____	_____

Supplements

YeastMAX – Candida Cleanse	30.00	_____	_____
ParaMAX – Parasite Cleanse	30.00	_____	_____
CleanseMAX – Bowel and Organ Cleansing	25.00	_____	_____
Barlean's Flax Seed Oil – 16 oz.	12.50	_____	_____
Barlean's Flax Seed Oil – 32 oz.	24.50	_____	_____
Barlean's Flax Seek Oil Capsules – 100 count	7.50	_____	_____
Ultra Pro Chocolate Protein Powder – 2 lbs.	49.00	_____	_____
Naturade Vegetable Protein Powder – 16 oz.	16.00	_____	_____
Designer Protein, Vanilla – 12 oz.	17.00	_____	_____
Designer Protein, Vanilla – 2 lbs.	36.00	_____	_____
Catalyst Multi-Vitamin & Mineral – 120 count	42.00	_____	_____
Trace Minerals Concentrace Mineral Drops – 4 oz.	13.50	_____	_____
Complete Calcium & Magnesium – 120 count	17.00	_____	_____
Unique E – 400 I.U. each – 90 count	23.00	_____	_____
PhytoBears – kid's phytonutrient supplement	19.50	_____	_____
Barlean's Greens – 9.3 oz. powder	31.00	_____	_____
ImmunoStart™ – colostrum, beta-1,3 / 1,6 glucans & lactoferrin	42.50	_____	_____
DSF – de-stress formula – 60 count	21.00	_____	_____
GlycoBears – children's multi-vitamin/mineral – 60 count chewables	22.00	_____	_____

Plus – wild yam/hormone support – 90 count		39.00	_____	_____
Natural Progesterone Cream		25.00	_____	_____
Natren Megadophilus – small intestine support		22.00	_____	_____
Natren Bifido – large intestine support		22.00	_____	_____
N-Zime #10 – general digestive enzyme support – 90 count		17.00	_____	_____
(Select Enzyme Solutions per Enzyme Questionairen on page 99.)				
Enzyme Solutions #1 – #36 (____ indicate #)		17.00	_____	_____
(All Enzyme Solutions prices are the same except the following.)				
Enzyme Solutions #17, #34 or #35 (____ indicate #)		30.00	_____	_____
Enzyme Solutions #33		40.00	_____	_____

Glyconutrients

Ambrotose Bulk Powder 100 grams – 8 month supply	125.00	_____	_____
Ambrotose Bulk Powder 50 grams – 4 month supply	69.00	_____	_____

Other

Blood Type Self Test Kit	15.00	_____	_____
Skin Brush – natural bristle	8.00	_____	_____
Shower Filter	49.00	_____	_____
Shower Filter Replacement Cartridge	25.00	_____	_____
Half-Fold Rebounder ($18 shipping fee)	249.00	_____	_____
Urban Rebounding Exercise Video	25.00	_____	_____
Bring Your Body to Life Exercise Program	99.00	_____	_____
_____	____.__	_____	_____
_____	____.__	_____	_____
_____	____.__	_____	_____
Complete Catalog and Product Order Information	Free	_____	_____
Skin Care Products Catalog and Order Information	Free	_____	_____

Shipping & Handling
$0 – $24.99 = $4.50
$25 – 80.99 = $6.00
$81 & up = $8.00
Large book orders will be sent UPS and billed based on weight.

Subtotal	_____
Shipping	_____
Tax (CO 3.8%)	_____
Total	_____

Charge to my ❑ Visa ❑ MasterCard ❑ American Express ❑ Personal Check

Card # _____ Expiration Date _____

Authorization Signature _____

Name _____

Address _____

City/State/Zip _____

Email _____

Home Phone _____ Fax _____ Work Phone _____

Mail Order to: Lifestyle for Health, 6520 S Broadway, Littleton, CO 80121, 303.794.4477

For Fastest Service fax your order to 303.794.1449 or order via the web at www.lifestyleforhealth.com.

Prices subject to change.

Lifestyle for Health Order Form

		Quantity	Total
Books			
Discovering Wholeness, Townsley	26.95	_____	_____
Food Smart!, Townsley	13.00	_____	_____
Kid Smart!, Townsley	15.00	_____	_____
Cleansing Made Simple, Townsley	10.00	_____	_____
Candida Simple, Townsley	12.00	_____	_____
Return to Paradise, Townsley	10.00	_____	_____
Healthy Habits, Frähm	13.00	_____	_____
Cookbooks			
Lifestyle for Health Cookbook, Townsley	26.00	1	_____
Meals in 30 Minutes, Townsley	15.00	1	_____
Candida Control Cookbook, Burton	14.00	_____	_____
Stevia Sweet Recipes, Goettemoeller	13.95	_____	_____
Audio Education			
Too Stressed to Be Blessed (4 tapes)	25.00	_____	_____
Raging Hormones (4 tapes)	25.00	_____	_____
Healthy Kids – Beating ADD (2 tapes)	15.00	_____	_____
Supplements – A Systems Approach (1 tape)	5.00	_____	_____
Health & Supplements on a Budget (1 tape)	5.00	_____	_____
Top 10 Health Builders & Busters (2 tapes w/notes)	20.00	_____	_____
Optimal Health Video	25.00	_____	_____
Skin Brushing the Gaither Way	30.00	_____	_____
Supplements			
YeastMAX – Candida Cleanse	30.00	_____	_____
ParaMAX – Parasite Cleanse	30.00	_____	_____
CleanseMAX – Bowel and Organ Cleansing	25.00	_____	_____
Barlean's Flax Seed Oil – 16 oz.	12.50	_____	_____
Barlean's Flax Seed Oil – 32 oz.	24.50	_____	_____
Barlean's Flax Seek Oil Capsules – 100 count	7.50	_____	_____
Ultra Pro Chocolate Protein Powder – 2 lbs.	49.00	_____	_____
Naturade Vegetable Protein Powder – 16 oz.	16.00	_____	_____
Designer Protein, Vanilla – 12 oz.	17.00	_____	_____
Designer Protein, Vanilla – 2 lbs.	36.00	_____	_____
Catalyst Multi-Vitamin & Mineral – 120 count	42.00	_____	_____
Trace Minerals Concentrace Mineral Drops – 4 oz.	13.50	_____	_____
Complete Calcium & Magnesium – 120 count	17.00	_____	_____
Unique E – 400 I.U. each – 90 count	23.00	_____	_____
PhytoBears – kid's phytonutrient supplement	19.50	_____	_____
Barlean's Greens – 9.3 oz. powder	31.00	_____	_____
ImmunoStart™ – colostrum, beta-1,3 / 1,6 glucans & lactoferrin	42.50	_____	_____
DSF – de-stress formula – 60 count	21.00	_____	_____
GlycoBears – children's multi-vitamin/mineral – 60 count chewables	22.00	_____	_____

Plus – wild yam/hormone support – 90 count	39.00	_____	_____
Natural Progesterone Cream	25.00	_____	_____
Natren Megadophilus – small intestine support	22.00	_____	_____
Natren Bifido – large intestine support	22.00	_____	_____
N-Zime #10 – general digestive enzyme support – 90 count	17.00	_____	_____
(Select Enzyme Solutions per Enzyme Questionairen on page 99.)			
Enzyme Solutions #1 – #36 (____ indicate #)	17.00	_____	_____
(All Enzyme Solutions prices are the same except the following.)			
Enzyme Solutions #17, #34 or #35 (____ indicate #)	30.00	_____	_____
Enzyme Solutions #33	40.00	_____	_____

Glyconutrients

Ambrotose Bulk Powder 100 grams – 8 month supply	125.00	_____	_____
Ambrotose Bulk Powder 50 grams – 4 month supply	69.00	_____	_____

Other

Blood Type Self Test Kit	15.00	_____	_____
Skin Brush – natural bristle	8.00	_____	_____
Shower Filter	49.00	_____	_____
Shower Filter Replacement Cartridge	25.00	_____	_____
Half-Fold Rebounder ($18 shipping fee)	249.00	_____	_____
Urban Rebounding Exercise Video	25.00	_____	_____
Bring Your Body to Life Exercise Program	99.00	_____	_____
_____	____.__	_____	_____
_____	____.__	_____	_____
_____	____.__	_____	_____
Complete Catalog and Product Order Information	Free	_____	_____
Skin Care Products Catalog and Order Information	Free	_____	_____

Shipping & Handling

    $0 – $24.99 = $4.50

    $25 – 80.99 = $6.00

    $81 & up = $8.00

    Large book orders will be sent UPS and billed based on weight.

Subtotal	_____
Shipping	_____
Tax (CO 3.8%)	_____
Total	_____

Charge to my ❑ Visa ❑ MasterCard ❑ American Express ❑ Personal Check

    Card # _____ Expiration Date _____

    Authorization Signature _____

    Name _____

    Address _____

    City/State/Zip _____

    Email _____

    Home Phone _____ Fax _____ Work Phone _____

Mail Order to: Lifestyle for Health, 6520 S Broadway, Littleton, CO 80121, 303.794.4477

For Fastest Service fax your order to 303.794.1449 or order via the web at www.lifestyleforhealth.com.

Prices subject to change.

Lifestyle for Health Order Form

		Quantity	Total

Books

Discovering Wholeness, Townsley	26.95	_____	_____
Food Smart!, Townsley	13.00	_____	_____
Kid Smart!, Townsley	15.00	_____	_____
Cleansing Made Simple, Townsley	10.00	_____	_____
Candida Simple, Townsley	12.00	_____	_____
Return to Paradise, Townsley	10.00	_____	_____
Healthy Habits, Frähm	13.00	_____	_____

Cookbooks

Lifestyle for Health Cookbook, Townsley	26.00	_____	_____
Meals in 30 Minutes, Townsley	15.00	_____	_____
Candida Control Cookbook, Burton	14.00	_____	_____
Stevia Sweet Recipes, Goettemoeller	13.95	_____	_____

Audio Education

Too Stressed to Be Blessed (4 tapes)	25.00	_____	_____
Raging Hormones (4 tapes)	25.00	_____	_____
Healthy Kids – Beating ADD (2 tapes)	15.00	_____	_____
Supplements – A Systems Approach (1 tape)	5.00	_____	_____
Health & Supplements on a Budget (1 tape)	5.00	_____	_____
Top 10 Health Builders & Busters (2 tapes w/notes)	20.00	_____	_____
Optimal Health Video	25.00	_____	_____
Skin Brushing the Gaither Way	30.00	_____	_____

Supplements

YeastMAX – Candida Cleanse	30.00	_____	_____
ParaMAX – Parasite Cleanse	30.00	_____	_____
CleanseMAX – Bowel and Organ Cleansing	25.00	_____	_____
Barlean's Flax Seed Oil – 16 oz.	12.50	_____	_____
Barlean's Flax Seed Oil – 32 oz.	24.50	_____	_____
Barlean's Flax Seek Oil Capsules – 100 count	7.50	_____	_____
Ultra Pro Chocolate Protein Powder – 2 lbs.	49.00	_____	_____
Naturade Vegetable Protein Powder – 16 oz.	16.00	_____	_____
Designer Protein, Vanilla – 12 oz.	17.00	_____	_____
Designer Protein, Vanilla – 2 lbs.	36.00	_____	_____
Catalyst Multi-Vitamin & Mineral – 120 count	42.00	_____	_____
Trace Minerals Concentrace Mineral Drops – 4 oz.	13.50	_____	_____
Complete Calcium & Magnesium – 120 count	17.00	_____	_____
Unique E – 400 I.U. each – 90 count	23.00	_____	_____
PhytoBears – kid's phytonutrient supplement	19.50	_____	_____
Barlean's Greens – 9.3 oz. powder	31.00	_____	_____
ImmunoStart™ – colostrum, beta-1,3 / 1,6 glucans & lactoferrin	42.50	_____	_____
DSF – de-stress formula – 60 count	21.00	_____	_____
GlycoBears – children's multi-vitamin/mineral – 60 count chewables	22.00	_____	_____

Plus – wild yam/hormone support – 90 count	39.00	_____	_____
Natural Progesterone Cream	25.00	_____	_____
Natren Megadophilus – small intestine support	22.00	_____	_____
Natren Bifido – large intestine support	22.00	_____	_____
N-Zime #10 – general digestive enzyme support – 90 count	17.00	_____	_____
(Select Enzyme Solutions per Enzyme Questionairen on page 99.)			
Enzyme Solutions #1 – #36 (____ indicate #)	17.00	_____	_____
(All Enzyme Solutions prices are the same except the following.)			
Enzyme Solutions #17, #34 or #35 (____ indicate #)	30.00	_____	_____
Enzyme Solutions #33	40.00	_____	_____

Glyconutrients

Ambrotose Bulk Powder 100 grams – 8 month supply	125.00	_____	_____
Ambrotose Bulk Powder 50 grams – 4 month supply	69.00	_____	_____

Other

Blood Type Self Test Kit	15.00	_____	_____
Skin Brush – natural bristle	8.00	_____	_____
Shower Filter	49.00	_____	_____
Shower Filter Replacement Cartridge	25.00	_____	_____
Half-Fold Rebounder ($18 shipping fee)	249.00	_____	_____
Urban Rebounding Exercise Video	25.00	_____	_____
Bring Your Body to Life Exercise Program	99.00	_____	_____
_____	____.__	_____	_____
_____	____.__	_____	_____
_____	____.__	_____	_____
Complete Catalog and Product Order Information	Free	_____	_____
Skin Care Products Catalog and Order Information	Free	_____	_____

Shipping & Handling	**Subtotal**	_____
$0 – $24.99 = $4.50	**Shipping**	_____
$25 – 80.99 = $6.00	**Tax** (CO 3.8%)	_____
$81 & up = $8.00	**Total**	_____
Large book orders will be sent UPS and billed based on weight.		

Charge to my ❑ Visa ❑ MasterCard ❑ American Express ❑ Personal Check

Card # _____ Expiration Date _____

Authorization Signature _____

Name _____

Address _____

City/State/Zip _____

Email _____

Home Phone _____ Fax _____ Work Phone _____

Mail Order to: Lifestyle for Health, 6520 S Broadway, Littleton, CO 80121, 303.794.4477

For Fastest Service fax your order to 303.794.1449 or order via the web at www.lifestyleforhealth.com.

Prices subject to change.